The International Library of Psychology

ON SHAME AND THE SEARCH FOR IDENTITY

Founded by C. K. Ogden

The International Library of Psychology

INDIVIDUAL DIFFERENCES
In 21 Volumes

I	The Practice and Theory of Individual Psychology	*Adler*
II	The Neurotic Constitution	*Adler*
III	Duality	*Bradley*
IV	Problems of Personality	*Campbell et al*
V	An Introduction to Individual Psychology	*Dreikurs*
VI	The Psychology of Alfred Adler and the Development of the Child	*Ganz*
VII	Personality	*Gordon*
VIII	The Art of Interrogation	*Hamilton*
IX	Appraising Personality	*Harrower*
X	Physique and Character	*Kretschmer*
XI	The Psychology of Men of Genius	*Kretschmer*
XII	Handreading	*Laffan*
XIII	On Shame and the Search for Identity	*Lynd*
XIV	A B C of Adler's Psychology	*Mairet*
XV	Alfred Adler: Problems of Neurosis	*Mairet*
XVI	Principles of Experimental Psychology	*Piéron*
XVII	The Psychology of Character	*Roback*
XVIII	The Hands of Children	*Spier*
XIX	The Nature of Intelligence	*Thurstone*
XX	Alfred Adler: The Pattern of Life	*Wolfe*
XXI	The Psychology of Intelligence and Will	*Wyatt*

ON SHAME AND THE SEARCH FOR IDENTITY

HELEN MERRELL LYND

Routledge
Taylor & Francis Group
LONDON AND NEW YORK

First published in 1958 by
Routledge
2 Park Square, Milton Park, Abingdon, Oxfordshire OX14 4RN
711 Third Avenue, New York, NY 10017

First issued in paperback 2014

Routledge is an imprint of the Taylor and Francis Group, an informa business

British Library Cataloguing in Publication Data
A CIP catalogue record for this book
is available from the British Library

On Shame and the Search for Identity
ISBN 0415-21063-1
Individual Differences: 21 Volumes
ISBN 0415-21130-1
The International Library of Psychology: 204 Volumes
ISBN 0415-19132-7

ISBN 13: 978-1-138-87542-5 (pbk)
ISBN 13: 978-0-415-21063-8 (hbk)

TO

my Students and Colleagues

Past and Present

at Sarah Lawrence College

Foreword

When should cumulating speculations on a subject be gathered together for publication? This book if published a year or two years from now would doubtless be different in many ways. But if it were not published for another ten years, it would still contain unresolved contradictions, and would take the form of questions and suggestions, not of final conclusions. One reason for publishing it now is to invite comment on the questions it raises.

The thought of a number of persons with whom I have discussed these questions over a period of years, including that of my son Staughton Lynd, is deeply woven into the entire book. More recently, I have had important criticisms on the manuscript before its final revision from Elizabeth Barnes, Robert K. Merton, David Riesman, and Lee R. Wolin. The usual disclaimer that much of the thought of others enters into whatever is of value in these pages but that the shortcomings are my own is more than usually relevant.

To Margaret Marshall I am doubly indebted. As Book Review Editor of *The Nation* she gave me an opportunity to do review articles that helped me to bring certain ideas into focus. On this book, she not only gave me valuable specific suggestions but had the imagination to create an atmosphere in which one's best work can be done.

Lucy Lowe has struggled with the typing of succeeding versions of this book. Her care and patience in this and in the preparation of the index have been invaluable.

HELEN MERRELL LYND

Sarah Lawrence College
January, 1958

Contents

On Shame and the Search for Identity

ONE

Introduction

Contemporary Search for Identity

In every age men ask in some form the questions: Who am I? Where do I belong? The degree of awareness and the kind of emphasis with which these questions are asked vary at different periods. Times of swift change and social dislocation bring them to the fore, against the background of whatever personal hopes and social harmonies an earlier period has cultivated.

Such times of change appear primarily as periods of dissolution or of new birth according to the particular view of individual values and historical sequences from which they are interpreted. To Burckhardt the Middle Ages was a time of "childish prepossession" happily succeeded by the "flowering of free personality" of the Renaissance. Other writers would single out other periods also in the history of the West as times of heightened awareness of individual identity: the transition from the age of Hesiod to fifth-century Greece and the period of the Hebrew prophets beginning in the seventh century,[a] the period of Plotinus, or of Rousseau, or of the nineteenth-century Romantics. Some would question Burckhardt's evaluation, and maintain that the insights of St. Augustine at the threshold of the Middle Ages held greater promise for the flowering of personality than the more exclusive forms of Renaissance ration-

[a] The notes begin on page 261.

alism. Whether in subsequent appraisals the stress falls on the loss of an earlier integration or on the shaping of new social forms, the individual man living through periods of transition is impelled to a fresh questioning of himself in relation to the world.

Certainly our own age is another such time. People of any period tend toward a kind of temporal centrism, which may be as confined in outlook as ethnocentrism. At present we may find it hard to believe that for St. Augustine or for Erasmus the discovery of identity was as important or as difficult as it is for us—just as we may learn with surprise that the coins of Hadrian in the first century were inscribed *Humanitas, Libertas, Felicitas.*

But whatever our limitations of outlook, it is manifest that the recurrent question of self-identity is today in the forefront of awareness. Today might be dated from the Copernican Revolution, from the Renaissance and the Reformation, from the French and Industrial revolutions, or from the First World War. I refer particularly to the last half, and especially the last quarter, century, when thinking people have had to attempt to assimilate the implications of an economy of potential abundance, of communication among all parts of the world, of colonial revolutions, world war, and concentration camps, of atomic energy, of the theories of Darwin, of Marx, of Freud, of Planck. Each of these historical developments has given our search for identity special possibilities, special difficulties, and our own peculiar version of its importance.

So great has been the impact of the changes of recent years that it is possible for an innovating Freudian psychoanalyst, Erik H. Erikson, to say that the search for identity has become as strategic in our time as the study of sexuality was in Freud's time. "The patient [or person] of today suffers most under the problem of what he should believe in and who he should—or, indeed, might—be or become; while the patient of early psychoanalysis suffered most under inhibitions which prevented him from being what and who he thought he knew he was." [a]

This search for identity, as will be apparent from all that follows, is a social as well as an individual problem. The kind of answer one gives to the question Who am I? depends in part upon how one answers the question What is this society—and this world—in which I live?

We might assume, on first thought, that if the question Who am I? is of particular importance at present, it is also receiving more than adequate attention as a matter of specialized study. Social scientists, psychologists and psychoanalysts of all schools, poets and novelists observe, describe, dissect, analyze, and bring the resources of technical skill and artistic insight to bear upon rediscovery of the meaning of individuality, upon the experiences of the individual in his attempt to attain a sense of himself and a place of anchorage in the world.

Above all, they *name* different aspects of these experiences. It is hard to find any phase of personality development or of social life that has not acquired a label with its rapidly codified weighting of association and meaning. The study of instincts may give way to the study of traits, and this, in turn, to the study of drives, motives, vectors, or variables as the terminology in favor changes; but it would seem that whatever the human experience, or aspect of personality, it could not escape being caught in the mesh of some scheme of codification.

Our period of history, too, is marked by self-conscious labels. It is called a new period of failure of nerve, an age of conformity, a period of *anomie* or cultural chaos, of escape from freedom, a new age of treason, an age of longing, a decline of the West. Much is heard of the dilemma of liberalism, the distrust of the democratic process, the revolt of the masses, the failure of self-determination, the loss of command over the environment. We who live in this time are described as alienated, estranged, isolated, alone, a lost generation, depersonalized, other-directed, double men.

However much we may question or qualify any particular label, there is a sense in which the fact of the labeling itself remains, in de Tocqueville's sense, a living witness to the concern with personal identity and social anchorage. The soberly academic statement "The child is born without an identity; he achieves one through his contact with the world around him," [a] and the darting insight "Life is . . . the oddest affair; has in it the essence of reality. I used to feel this as a child—couldn't step across a puddle once, I remember, for thinking how strange

—what am I?" [a]—each bears the peculiar mark not of any time, but of our time.

Elaboration of research methods in psychology and social science has kept pace with the proliferation of labeling. Observations, categories, techniques for the study of human nature were never so abundant; there were never so many people engaged in using them. If understanding of identity and of ways of realizing it could be discovered by such means, this strategic problem of today would seem assured of solution.

But since every way of seeing is also a way of not seeing, it is possible that the very multiplication of categories and the very precision of techniques may sometimes act as barriers instead of as means of access to understanding. Reliance on accepted categories and methods may mean that certain phenomena essential for understanding identity escape attention. In the present climate of psychological thought any observed human characteristic speedily acquires a label, which encases it within one of the experimentalists' or the clinicians' categories. Extensive as these categories are, applied to some life situations they may be more constricting than informing.

Certain pervasive experiences, not easily labeled, may slip through the categories altogether or, if given a location and a name, may be circumscribed in such a way that their essential character is lost. Habituation to such usage may blind us still further to the necessity of searching more deeply into the nature of these experiences.

Among such experiences are the diffused sensations of early childhood,[b] and other experiences that may occur in some form at many stages of life—shame, anxiety, joy, love, sense of honor, wonder, curiosity, longing, certain kinds of pride, self-respect. Of these, only anxiety has been the subject of extensive specialized study. (I do not include guilt among these pervasive phenomena for reasons that will appear later.) Such experiences tend to elude codification whether of the experimentalist's laboratory or of the psychoanalyst's schema. They are inaccessible to certain kinds of methods of precision. Since certain of these experiences, which are hard to isolate and confine, have a peculiarly close relation to the sense of identity it is important to look at them more carefully, both in a personal search for identity and in an effort to gain greater theoretical understanding of what identity means.

In these pages I shall attempt tentative exploration of one such experience—shame—familiar in name but far from clear in meaning. Most psychologists would agree that the cluster of phenomena roughly described as shame needs further study. There would be less agreement on the nature of these phenomena or with the suggestion that some of our current assumptions and methods in psychology and social science tend to block understanding of them.

I became interested in experiences of shame through coming to recognize that concepts of guilt as they are currently used, under a variety of names, are inadequate to explain certain types of experience and certain types of personality which they are assumed to include. They and their derivatives, moreover, leave much of the sense of identity unexplained and perhaps unexplainable. It then occurred to me that further exploration of experiences of shame might help to explain some neglected aspects of personality development and lead toward greater understanding of a sense of identity.

At this point I shall mention only briefly some of the things that drew my attention to differences between what I may call the guilt-axis and the shame-axis interpretations of personality.* The elaboration of these and of other aspects of guilt and shame as they are related to developing a sense of identity is the substance of this book.

The concept of guilt is much used at present as a general interpretation of the human situation. Protestant theologians such as Reinhold Niebuhr and Anglo-Catholics such as T. S. Eliot believe that the attempt to substitute an optimistic humanitarianism for man's consciousness of guilt is one of the reasons for the present plight of the world. Freudians and some existentialists believe that a sense of guilt pervades life and is one of man's tragedies. They debate among themselves as to whether this feeling of guilt is particularly characteristic of heirs to the Puritan tradition, of Western society, or of all humanity.

* These two interpretations or emphases, as will appear in the following discussion, are not mutually exclusive but complementary.

Although the concept of guilt is prevalent in philosophical explanations of man's lot, contemporary methods of child rearing, of teaching, of social counseling—except perhaps in some religious groups—do not ostensibly attempt to develop and make use of a sense of guilt. Terms associated with guilt have tended to be dropped as inciters to desirable action. Sophisticated parents, teachers, or therapists no longer say that a child is good or bad. But the words good and bad have been replaced by mature and immature, productive and unproductive, socially adjusted and maladjusted. And when these words are used by the teacher, the counselor, or the therapist they carry the same weight of approbation and disapprobation as the earlier good and bad. The prescriptions for being mature are as specific as the earlier prescriptions for being good. It is mature to handle money and work effectively, to adjust to reality, to take responsibility, to be decisive in action, to make vocational choices commensurate with one's ability, to be successful in what one undertakes, to use leisure productively, to have friends of both sexes, to have at the appropriate age heterosexual relations. This is being mature in terms of the demands of what is variously described as the achievement, performance, or success norms or the market-place psychology of our contemporary society.[a] (I am not now questioning specifically any of these criteria; I am simply pointing out that together they constitute as rigid a code as that of any church or creed.) The reverse of these things is immature or bad; and an individual feels the appropriate guilt if he does not attain maturity in the prescribed manner. Adjustment in terms of the realities of our present society sometimes appears to have replaced hope of heaven as the supreme good.

But one may follow all the precepts laid down by teachers, social scientists, social workers, and psychoanalysts and still feel that something is lacking—that the central core of the self is untouched. On the other hand, one may transgress no code, commit no proscribed act, meet all the standards of society and of the experts in personality and yet feel a meanness or inadequacy which violates the core of oneself. This is truer for some people than for others; for some the codes of mature adjustment and the purposes of the self more nearly coincide.

It was this impression of the insufficiency of the guilt-axis interpretation of personality, by whatever name it goes, that sent me searching for other possible ways of approaching personal identity, for other concepts and emphases that might more fully account for some experiences and for some people.

It was when I began to search for significant experiences omitted by interpretations based on the guilt axis alone, and for other ways of approaching the development of the sense of self, that it occurred to me that experiences of shame are relatively little studied and that they might offer important clues for the understanding of the sense of identity. They are obviously only one source of such clues, but I thought they might prove to be a particularly significant one. With all our apparatus of psychological investigation, shame is relatively little studied because in our society it is so easily linked with or subsumed under guilt. The questions of why it is so early absorbed by guilt in our society and why our methods of inquiry lead us more readily to the study of guilt than of shame invite further consideration.

The word shame—or talk of being ashamed of ourselves—does not occur as frequently in conversation today as it did, for example, in the conversations of Tolstoy's characters. We do not verbally "shame" our children, although in less obvious ways we may make them ashamed. We strive for self-enlightenment, we attempt to accept the limitations of ourselves and of reality, and to live up to the standards derived from therapy and from theories of social adjustment.* These "realistic" emphases may tend to keep us from confronting shame.

But it is doubtful whether the sense of shame has disappeared from actual experience to the extent that it has disappeared from our speech and from the forefront of our consciousness. It may be that the experience is no less common than at some other periods but that it is more elusive and that we are more loath to recognize it.

It is no accident that experiences of shame are called *self*-consciousness. Such experiences are characteristically painful. They are usually taken as something to be hidden, dodged, cov-

* These do not always coincide. There are some psychoanalysts who do not make social adjustment central in therapy.

ered up—even, or especially, from oneself. Shame interrupts any unquestioning, unaware sense of oneself. But it is possible that experiences of shame if confronted full in the face may throw an unexpected light on who one is and point the way toward who one may become. Fully faced, shame may become not primarily something to be covered, but a positive experience of revelation.

In this first chapter I shall deal briefly with the derivations and usages of the two words shame and guilt. In the next chapter I shall attempt a more detailed description of experiences of shame. The third chapter will examine some of the assumptions that underlie prevailing methods of study in psychology and social science which lead to the neglect of such a pervasive experience as shame and its absorption into guilt in contemporary study. The fourth will examine some newer methods coming into use which may throw more light on experiences such as shame and the sense of identity. The final chapter will explore the implications and point the meaning of the preceding discussion for the development of a sense of identity.

Discussion of these questions in the third and fourth chapters involves dealing with the materials and methods of psychology and of the social sciences. The aim, however, is not appraisal of these different areas of study, but seeing—in regard to the experiences of shame and identity—what light these disciplines can throw on the nature of human beings, of their relations to each other, and of their relations to the world. These might be called essentially questions of philosophy, or of social philosophy. It has always been the function of philosophy to push questions beyond accepted barriers. In doing so it has always inevitably made use of what can be learned from more specialized fields of study.

The Concepts Shame and Guilt

The reason for considering meanings associated with the word shame is not to engage in a linguistic exercise but to discover a possible clue to the experience. From the outset we encounter difficulties about the meaning of the word. Although it may have somewhat dropped out of popular usage, it appears frequently in social science and psychological discussion. But it carries no clear or consistent meaning. Often it is coupled with guilt, and the phrase "shame and guilt" is used as if it were one descriptive term. Again, and sometimes by the same persons who use this coupling phrase, shame and guilt are contrasted in ways that have become widespread conventions. Thus Freud says that self-reproach (for a sexual act in childhood) can easily become shame lest another person should hear about it.[a] Guilt, or self-reproach, is based on internalization of values, notably parental values—in contrast to shame, which is based upon disapproval coming from outside, from other persons. Ruth Benedict makes a similar distinction. She contrasts guilt, a failure to live up to one's own picture of oneself (based on parental values), with shame, a reaction to criticism by other people.[b]

This distinction between guilt and shame—as oriented respectively to oneself through the internalization of identifications with one's parents and to others through their expressed ridicule or scorn—has been until recently the basis of the most widely accepted definitions of the two terms.[c]

Involved in this distinction between guilt as response to standards that have been internalized and shame as response to criticism or ridicule by others are several important assumptions, sometimes made explicit but more often unstated by the persons who use them: that shame is a more external experience than guilt, one that does not exist apart from the expressed scorn of other persons, if not in their actual presence; that there is a basic separation between oneself and others; that others are related to oneself as audience—whether the audience gives approval or disapproval.

Although the distinctions between shame and guilt that Freud and Benedict made are still those most commonly accepted by writers who use the two concepts, these distinctions and the assumptions that have led to them are beginning to be questioned. Among some psychoanalysts and social scientists there is recognition that important differences may be confused and that certain aspects of shame may be neglected altogether if current usage in distinguishing it from guilt is followed.

The different attempts to discover other and possibly more fruitful ways of describing experiences of shame and guilt do not discard insights gained from earlier formulations. Rather, they call attention to neglected aspects of these experiences and point toward a variety of other ways of approaching them. These recent suggestions include distinctions: between the content of the experience (what it is about which one feels shame or guilt) and the source of the disapproval (primarily oneself or primarily other persons);[a] between the forbidding and the sanctioning or goal-creating aspects of what Freud called the superego;[b] between the feeling of inferiority and the feeling of wrongdoing;[c] between feelings of inferiority for not meeting standards set by the culture and feelings of inferiority in relation to values that are wider than those of a particular culture.[d]

One of the most interesting of the recent formulations of the differences between shame and guilt is that of Gerhart Piers. In Piers' view the crucial distinction between guilt and shame is not that between self-criticism and criticism by others but between transgression of prohibitions and failure to reach goals or ideals.

> Whereas guilt is generated whenever a boundary . . . is touched or transgressed, shame occurs when a goal . . . is not being reached. It thus indicates a real "shortcoming." Guilt anxiety accompanies transgression; shame, failure.[e]

A somewhat similar distinction is made by Franz Alexander. Guilt, he believes, gives rise to the feeling "I am no good" in contrast to the feeling in shame "I am weak" or inadequate. A sense of guilt arises from a feeling of wrongdoing, a sense of shame from a feeling of inferiority. Inferiority feelings in shame are rooted in a deeper conflict in the personality than the sense of wrongdoing in guilt; feelings of inferiority, in this view, are presocial phenomena, whereas guilt feelings result from efforts for social adjustment.[f]

It is implied by the recent approaches from different directions to experiences of shame and guilt that the same situation may give rise to both shame and guilt; that shame and guilt may sometimes alternate with and reinforce each other;[g] and that a particular situation may be experienced by an individual as shame or guilt or both according to the nature of the person, the axis on which he habitually behaves, and the nature of his relation to other persons who may be involved. Shame and guilt are in no sense—either in the older or in the more recent conceptions of the experiences—antitheses, or at opposite poles from each other. Rather, they involve different focuses, modes, and stresses. Often they overlap, and it is partly for this reason that the study of shame has been subsumed under, or neglected in, the study of guilt.

The importance of reconsideration of the meaning of shame does not, as noted above, lie in the redefining of a particular word. The question is whether customary definitions and usage have led to the neglect of significant experiences that may be of special relevance for the understanding of identity. Goethe once remarked that the greatest difficulty about a problem lay in where one did not search for it. It is the sense of the importance of shame as an area where one should search that has led me to this further exploration.

The word shame has a long history in the nontheoretical, literary record of human experience. Both shame and guilt derive from Old English roots; but shame appears in some form in all Germanic languages, while there is no cognate word for guilt in other languages. The root meaning of shame is to cover up, to envelop; in some languages, as in much literary association, it also carries the meaning of wound. The Old English root of guilt carries the double meaning of guilt and debt.

Through all the root meanings of guilt runs something that corresponds closely to Piers' conception. Guilt is centrally a transgression, a crime, the violation of a specific taboo, boundary, or legal code by a definite voluntary act. Through the various shadings of meaning there is the sense of the committing of a specific offense, the state of being justifiably liable to penalty. In the usual definitions there is no self-reference as there is in shame.

Both the Freud-Benedict and the Piers conceptions of shame go far back in the meaning of the word. Like honor, shame is a multifaceted word. It includes the subjective feeling of the person and the objective nature of the act. Shame is defined as a wound to one's self-esteem, a painful feeling or sense of degradation excited by the consciousness of having done something unworthy of one's previous idea of one's own excellence. It is, also, a peculiarly painful feeling of being in a situation that incurs the scorn or contempt of others. The awareness of self is central in both conceptions, but in the second the feeling or action of others is also a part of shame. There is no legal reference as in guilt, no question of a failure to pay a debt, and less implication of the violation of a prescribed code.

English and German each have one word for shame (shame in English, *Scham* in German) that combines the meanings of shame in one's own eyes with shame in the eyes of others. German reflects the self-reference of shame and the external obligation implied in guilt: *Ich schäme mich,* but *Ich bin schuldig.** *Schuldig,* guilty, means also owing a debt, duty, or obligation.

French and classical Greek each have two words for shame, connoting respectively its more private and its more public aspects.[a] *Pudeur* in French is associated particularly with the covering up of sex; it is modesty, bashfulness. *Honte* adds to these disgrace, a loss of honor in the eyes of others. *Pudeur* may keep one from an act; *honte* may be felt after an act.[b]

Aidos as used by Homer made little distinction between private and public shame; between respect for gods and for custom. Later, *aischyne* was differentiated from *aidos*. *Aidos* continued to be what one felt when confronted with the things nature tells one to revere not violate, such as shame related to sexual matters. *Aischyne* was associated with dishonor, with the emphasis on man-made codes. *Aidos* linked shame to awe.[c]

Further insight into the different associations carried by the words guilt and shame comes from the very different meanings of guiltless and shameless. Guiltless is quite clearly an honorific term. To be guiltless is to be free from guilt, innocent, blameless. Shameless, however, is a term of opprobrium. To be shameless is to be insensible to one's self; it is to be lacking in shame, unblushing, brazen, incorrigible.

> The unjust knoweth no shame.[d]

* A similar distinction is reflected in German between anxiety and fear: *Ich ängste mich* but *Ich fürchte etwas.*

As you were past all shame,—
Those of your fact are so,—so past all truth[a]

A wisp of straw were worth a thousand crowns
To make this shameless callet know herself.[b]

In the courts of Attica the defendant had his place beside a stone dedicated to *aidos;* the stone of the prosecutor on the opposite side was dedicated to *anaideia,* shamelessness. The one was entitled to conceal, the other obliged to unmask.[c]

The word guilt occurs twice in the Old Testament,[d] and guiltiness occurs twice,[e] neither is found in the New Testament. Both are associated with the shedding of blood. Guilty is used in the sense of having committed a crime. Guiltless is always used in the sense of innocent.

Shame appears frequently in both the Old and New Testaments. It is contrasted with glory.

. . . how long will ye turn my glory into shame?[f]

Whose end is destruction, whose God is their belly, and whose glory is in their shame.[g]

It is associated with confounding and confusion.

Let them be ashamed and confounded together that seek after my soul to destroy it; let them be driven backward and put to shame.[h]

Shame is also associated with covering the face.

We are confounded, because we have heard reproach; shame hath covered our faces.[i]

Acceptance of shame is the ultimate in commitment.

. . . rejoicing that they were accounted worthy to suffer shame for his name.[j]

Jesus . . . who for the joy that was set before him endured the cross, despising the shame. . . .[k]

Shakespeare uses shame about nine times as often as guilt.[l] Guilty, guiltiness, guiltless, and other derivatives are used altogether slightly more than the various derivatives of shame, including shamed, shameful, shameless, shamefaced, and its other form, shamefast. Shame is contrasted not with right-doing, nor with approval by others, but with truth and honor.

> And I can teach thee, coz, to shame the devil
> By telling truth. "Tell truth and shame the devil."
> If thou have power to raise him, bring him hither,
> And I'll be sworn I have power to shame him hence.
> O, while you live, tell truth and shame the devil! [a]

> Thou dost shame thy mother
> and wound her honour with this diffidence.[b]

> So shall my virtue be his vice's bawd;
> And he shall spend mine honour with his shame,
> As thriftless sons their scraping fathers' gold.
> Mine honour lives when his dishonour dies,
> Or my sham'd life in his dishonour lies.[c]

> No more my King, for he dishonours me,
> But most himself if he could see his shame.[d]

> I do shame
> To think of what a noble strain you are,
> And of how coward a spirit.[e]

In the same way that both the wounding of one's own self-ideal and disgrace in the eyes of others inhere in conceptions of shame, so, also, does honor include the contrasting meanings of self-realization which may be unknown to others and of public acclaim. To Hotspur honor embodies the chivalric ideal of personal glory in the eyes of others, a view that Falstaff's speech on honor echoes. But to Prince Hal honor is more than renown, or outward show in the eyes of men; as long as he has proved himself worthy in his own eyes he cares nothing for recognition from others.[f] This is the counterpart of shame.

The association of the word shame with loss of honor and of self-respect suggests why shame may be felt as something different from the guilt involved in failure to pay a debt, in violation of a prohibition, or in transgression of a boundary. The close association of shame with the self suggests also why further study of experiences of shame may lead to more understanding of the meaning of identity.

TWO

The Nature of Shame

In this chapter I shall attempt to enter further into the nature of the feeling of shame. I am not trying to build up any logical, or perhaps even consistent, definition of shame. Rather, I shall approach the feeling of shame from different directions and in different ways, and present situations that have been described by various writers as giving rise to a sense of shame. This assumes that there are some common characteristics of the feelings of shame that may occur in a variety of circumstances, and possibly some common characteristics among these diverse circumstances.

The different aspects or characteristics of shame, mentioned separately for purposes of examination, are so intermeshed with each other that each can be fully perceived and understood only within the context of the whole experience.

Exposure, Particularly Unexpected Exposure

Experiences of shame appear to embody the root meaning of the word—to uncover, to expose, to wound. They are experiences of exposure, exposure of peculiarly sensitive, intimate, vulnerable aspects of the self.* The exposure may be to others

* See pp. 166-71, 204-07 for the different ways in which the terms self, ego, and personality are used.

but, whether others are or are not involved, it is always, as will be shown more fully below, exposure to one's own eyes.

The particular aspects of the self especially vulnerable to exposure differ in different cultures.* Adam and Eve felt shame in becoming aware of their own nakedness. Throughout our Western civilization shame is related to the uncovering of nakedness. The terms *Scham* and *Schamgefühl* in German carry the implication of uncovered nudity, and *Scham* is part of the compound words referring particularly to the genitals.

In other societies shame may be more related to exposure while eating, to exposure of certain kinds of contact with kinfolk or with certain kinfolk, to exposure in initiation ceremonies or other stylized rituals surrounded with special sanctions, and to a whole range of patterns of social intercourse and social custom that it does not occur to us to cover up. This would suggest that there is a recognizable feeling of shame that arises in different societies, although the particular aspects of the self related to that feeling and the situations that give rise to it differ widely from one society to another.

Even within our own Western society there are wide individual differences as to what it is most shameful to have uncovered. For Philip in *Of Human Bondage*[a] it was his clubfoot, still more his feeling about allowing it to be exposed. For Virginia Woolf it was her writing and her ability, as a writer, to stand aside and observe the misery of others: "Is the time ever coming when I can endure to read my own writing in print without blushing—shivering and wishing to take cover?"[b] For Rousseau it was his lie accusing the maid of having stolen Mademoiselle Pontal's ribbon, which he himself had stolen.[c] For Kitty in *Anna Karenina* it was the open exposure of her love for

* The terms culture and society are sometimes used by anthropologists and other social scientists as virtually synonymous, and writers who do differentiate them have no common usage. I use the two terms in this book in ways that do not require fine distinctions between them. In general, I use society for the organized institutions of a social group that constitute its functioning and provide for its survival as a group; culture for the shared, learned traditions of a group that are passed on from one generation to the next. But in some places it seems appropriate to use culture in the wider anthropological sense that includes both the functioning society and its traditions.

Vronsky which was unreturned;[a] for Anna herself it was the secret recognition within herself of her love for Vronsky.[b] Dmitri Karamazov, on trial for murdering his father, suffered his greatest misery at having to take off his socks.

They were very dirty . . . and now everyone could see it. And what was worse he disliked his feet. All his life he had thought both his big toes hideous. He particularly loathed the coarse, flat, crooked nail on the right one, and now they would all see it. Feeling intolerably ashamed . . .[c]

Not wholly dissimilar was the experience of Mr. Pinkerton, the gray little amateur detective. All his life ashamed of penury, he preferred to be hanged for murder rather than to produce his alibi which would have involved the admission of mousy economy—that he had gone to a sixpenny rather than a shilling washroom. Freud pointed out that in some people shame may be excited less by feelings associated specifically with sex than by certain other feelings one is loath to admit to oneself.[d]

Closer examination of some of these experiences raises further questions about the nature of shame. For Rousseau, as for Dmitri Karamazov and for Mr. Pinkerton, exposure or fear of exposure to other persons certainly added to the sense of shame. But I think that this public exposure of even a very private part of one's physical or mental character could not in itself have brought about shame unless one had already felt within oneself, not only dislike, but shame for these traits. It is also true that if one discovered that one was not alone in having these traits shame would in one sense be alleviated by being shared; but if one still felt these characteristics as mean and ugly no matter how many people had them, shame would in another sense be extended.*

Philip's exposure of his clubfoot also raises the question of the relation of exposure to others and to oneself. After the school bully had twisted his arm until Philip put his foot out of bed to let the boys see his clubfoot

Philip . . . had got his teeth in the pillow so that his sobbing should be inaudible. He was not crying for the pain they had caused

* Cf. discussion of shame for others, pp. 53-63.

him, nor for the humiliation he had suffered when they looked at his foot, but with rage at himself because, unable to stand the torture, he had put out his foot of his own accord.[a]

Exposure to others was less painful to Philip than the exposure to himself of his own weakness. This incident also raises the questions, discussed later, of the extent to which an experience of shame is the result of a voluntary action which one brings on oneself or something which comes on one from without, and of the importance of the element of the unexpected in shame. Both deliberate and involuntary action may be involved. Maugham does not say whether the yielding to pain came suddenly for Philip. But it is more than possible that the final giving in and showing of his foot was unexpected, and that each time it occurred it had an element of surprise as if it had happened wholly against his will.

Anna Karenina lays bare wide varieties of shame experienced by very different kinds of people. In all of them, though other persons are sometimes present and involved, it is the exposure of oneself to oneself that is crucial. No one but Anna knew of her feelings as she recalled her encounters with Vronsky.

> [On the train returning from Moscow she] reviewed all her memories of her visit . . . they were all pleasant and good. She remembered the ball, she remembered Vronsky . . . she recalled all her relations with him; there was nothing to be ashamed of. But at the same time in these reminiscences the sense of shame kept growing stronger and stronger . . . that inward voice, whenever she thought of Vronsky, seemed to say: "Warmly, very warmly, passionately." [b]

No one but Anna knew of the unmerited sharp reproof she gave to her dressmaker, nor of the shame it brought to her because she knew it resulted from her thoughts of Vronsky.[c] The shame that Anna and Vronsky felt after their first intercourse was shame that each felt differently and that was unshared.

> . . . There was something horrible and revolting [to each of them] in the memory of what had been bought at this fearful price of shame. The shame in the presence of their physical nakedness crushed her and took hold of him.[d]

It was Anna alone who knew of her shame and alarm "at the new spiritual condition in which she found herself. She felt as though everything were beginning to be double in her soul." [a]

Levin felt not only the shame of rejection by Kitty, these "wounds that never healed," but also the shame known only to himself that followed a "fall" from chastity.[b] (This last is similar to the shame Philip felt in showing his clubfoot, a deliberate act which was, nevertheless, each time unexpected.) Kitty, recalling painfully to herself a year later the loving glance she had cast at Vronsky at the ball, said that she had acted "worse than badly,—shamefully." [c]

Dostoevski, who knew so many hidden aspects of shame, recognized that the deepest shame is exposure to oneself even though no one else may pay any attention to or even know of it.

> Even in forty years I would remember with loathing and humiliation those filthiest, most ludicrous, and most awful moments in my life. No one could have gone out of his way to degrade himself more shamelessly.[d]

The Scarlet Letter, an unfolding of shame, does not fail to note that the deepest shame is not shame in the eyes of others but weakness in one's own eyes. Public exposure may even be a protection against this more painful inner shame. Dimmesdale said, "Happy are you, Hester, that wear the scarlet letter openly upon your bosom! Mine burns in secret!" [e] This raises the question of when public knowledge re-enforces and when it is an easing of shame known to oneself.

However much schools of psychoanalysis may differ in their explanations of fear of exposure, shame, humiliation, there can be no doubt of the extent to which shame operates in the analytic hour, nor of the intensification of shame if there is a lack of understanding, or any sign of contempt, on the part of the analyst. But, here again, shame is the outcome not only of exposing oneself to another person but of the exposure to oneself of parts of the self that one has not recognized and whose existence one is reluctant to admit.

There is a particularly deep shame in deceiving other persons into believing something about oneself that is not true.

No one else knows of it; one has lied to oneself. This comes about in part because one doesn't know how to fit shame into the network of other emotions with which it is interwoven. It is closely associated with anger and bitterness, emotions that according to our code should be repressed, and may be turned against the self. Not knowing what should be done with shame one's first impulse is to conceal it, and this may produce further shame.

The exposure to oneself is at the heart of shame. In reviewing Stendhal's *Diaries,* Auden expressed surprise that Stendhal found it hard to admit certain things to himself and asked, "How can admitting anything to oneself be daring?" [a] In raising this remarkable question Auden reflects the extent to which many people at present have become insensitive to the experience of shame and to the deep ambiguities in human nature in which it is rooted.

More than other emotions, shame involves a quality of the unexpected; if in any way we feel it coming we are powerless to avert it. This is in part because of the difficulty we have in admitting to ourselves either shame or the circumstances that give rise to shame. Whatever part voluntary action may have in the experience of shame is swallowed up in the sense of something that overwhelms us from without and "takes us" unawares. We are taken by surprise, caught off guard, or off base, caught unawares, made a fool of. It is as if we were suddenly invaded from the rear where we cannot see, are unprotected, and can be overpowered.[b]

Kafka's *The Trial* is a study of the shame and bewilderment that may come from being taken by surprise, unprepared. "One is so unprepared," says K. He felt "the shame of being delivered into the hands of these people by his sudden weakness." " 'I don't know this law,' said K"; ". . . this unexpected question confused the man, which was the more deeply embarrassing as he was obviously a man of the world"; "One day—quite unexpectedly—some Judge will take up the documents . . . and order an immediate arrest." [c]

As in the case of Philip's suddenly giving in and showing his clubfoot, the phenomenon of unexpected yielding to physical and mental torture has been observed in the extreme conditions of concentration camps when persons felt the shame of being helpless and defeated, of being betrayed by their own bodies and minds.[a] ". . . victims of the Nazi inquisition have [said] that the moment of surrender occurred suddenly and against their will. For days they had faced the fury of their interrogators, and then suddenly they fell apart. 'All right, all right, you can have anything you want.' "[b]

Blushing manifests the exposure, the unexpectedness, the involuntary nature of shame. One's feeling is involuntarily exposed openly in one's face; one is uncovered. With blushing comes the impulse to "cover one's face," "bury one's face," "sink into the ground." "When the heart's past hope the face is past shame," says a Scottish proverb.

This association of shame with involuntary exposure of the face appears in both the Old and the New Testaments.

They looked unto him, and were lightened: and their faces were not ashamed.[c]

[I] said, O my God, I am ashamed and blush to lift up my face to thee . . .[d]

Were they ashamed when they had committed abomination? Nay, they were not at all ashamed, neither could they blush . . .[e]

Shakespeare associates changes of color in the face with the uncovering of shame.

> No, Plantagenet,
> 'Tis not for fear but anger that thy cheeks
> Blush for pure shame to counterfeit our roses,
> And yet thy tongue will not confess thy error.[f]

> Thou changed and self-cover'd thing, for shame!
> Bemonster not thy feature![g]

Different as are the varieties of shame experienced by the different persons in *Anna Karenina,* all are accompanied by blushing.

"My words must make a deep impression on you, since you remember them so well," said Levin, and, suddenly conscious that he had said just the same thing before, he grew red in the face.[a]

"Oh, [my husband] doesn't even know," [Anna] said, and suddenly a hot flush came over her face; her cheeks, her brow, her neck crimsoned, and tears of shame came into her eyes.[b]

On seeing [Anna, her husband] would have risen, but changed his mind, then his face flushed hotly—for the first time since Anna had known him he blushed, and he got up quickly and went to meet her, looking not at her eyes, but above them at her forehead and hair.[c]

The feeling of unexpectedness marks one of the central contrasts between shame and guilt. This unexpectedness is more than suddenness in time; it is also an astonishment at seeing different parts of ourselves, conscious and unconscious, acknowledged and unacknowledged, suddenly coming together, and coming together with aspects of the world we have not recognized.[d] Patterns of events (inner and outer) of which we are not conscious come unexpectedly into relation with those of which we are aware. In situations in which we feel guilty, choice, foresight, awareness in regard to a specific act are at least possible. Being taken unpleasantly by surprise, the impossibility of ordered behavior, the sudden sense of exposure, of being unable to deal with what is happening, characterize shame. It is as if a self of which we were not aware makes us unable to grasp the situation and to control what we do. In shame, says Erikson, one is conscious of being—when one is unprepared—exposed, looked at, all around.[e]

Incongruity or Inappropriateness

Being taken unawares is shameful when what is suddenly exposed is incongruous with, or glaringly inappropriate to, the situation, or to our previous image of ourselves in it.* There is

* Not all being taken unawares is shameful, and not all incongruity is shameful. Delight may come upon us unexpectedly and may be enhanced by elements of incongruity. Unexpectedness and incongruity are, nevertheless, essential elements in shame.

nothing *wrong* with what we have done; no sin has been committed. But discrepancy appears between us and the social situation, between what we feel from within and what appears to us, and perhaps to others, seen from without.* We have acted on the assumption of being one kind of person living in one kind of surroundings, and unexpectedly, violently, we discover that these assumptions are false. We had thought that we were able to see around certain situations and, instead, discover in a moment that it is we who are exposed; alien people in an alien situation can see around us.

Bernard Shaw believed that men are never at home in society, that they remain in a false position until "they have realized their possibilities. . . . They are tormented by a continual shortcoming in themselves; yet they irritate others by a continual overweening. . . . This finding of one's place may be made very puzzling by the fact that there is no place in ordinary society for extraordinary individuals." [a] Extraordinary individuals might include, in a sense wider than Shaw's, deviant, or innovating, or revolutionary, as well as markedly creative and independent individuals.

The attempt to understand experiences of being suddenly out of key with one's environment, and the recognition that such experiences may occur more often and more acutely for exceptional, or, as Shaw says, for extraordinary, individuals raises a question, suggested earlier, that should be borne in mind throughout this discussion: Does the feeling of shame imply an acceptance of the validity† of the values or standards of the society in relation to which one feels ashamed? Or, may there be personal or widely human values (if not standards) not wholly derived from the culture, in terms of which one judges not only oneself but one's society as well?

My tentative hypothesis is that the second comes closer to the truth, that aspects of the phenomenon of shame can be understood only with reference to transcultural values, and that

* See pp. 204-07 on the double direction of identity.

† Acceptance of legitimacy of standards should be distinguished from acceptance of their validity. One may recognize that certain things are required by law without believing that the laws are valid.

this awareness of values beyond one's own society is one of the distinctions between shame and guilt.

This statement needs immediate qualification, and it is not easy to state this view exactly, still less to substantiate it. If a person were wholly independent of the demands and conventions of his society, he might not feel shame, but the feeling of shame for the values of one's society, and the transcending of personal shame, would seem to depend upon having some perspective, some standards of significance, against which one can call into question the codes of one's immediate culture. The occasion for the comparison and the feeling of the need for it may arise out of a situation of shame in which there was initially no separate awareness of the values of one's culture as something to be questioned against the perspective of wider values. Some latent readiness to recognize this wider perspective must, however, have been present. Huckleberry Finn's conscience persistently nagged him because he did not report the Negro Jim, a runaway slave. According to the only moral code he had been taught, Jim was Miss Watson's property, and he ought to paddle ashore and tell someone that Jim was almost free. His guilt was compounded when he heard Jim talk of buying or stealing his children, who were the property of another owner. Huckleberry Finn had no doubt that he was doing wrong, but, because of some wider feeling of human decency that he could not name, he could not bring himself to do what his society called right.[a] The distinctions that some psychologists and philosophers have made between social codes and sources of shame beyond the moral codes of any society cannot be ignored, and these distinctions invite further exploration.[b] Complete cultural relativism need not be regarded as either as simple or as final as it was held to be by many people when it first provided a valuable corrective to ideas of absolute or authoritarian moral values. Never losing sight of the extent to which standards and values are the result of a particular upbringing in a particular society, we can now begin the exploration of common human desires, decencies, and values—and of the variety and richness of human values—that may be appealed to beyond those that are shaped by particular societies or particular cultural traditions.

The possibility of transcultural values is a highly complex question, which will be approached in different ways in what follows. It involves selective identification with different aspects of one's culture, and the individual combining of these selected aspects into new forms as well as identifications with wider values beyond those of one's immediate culture.[a] It also involves the distinction between feeling shame for things that one believes one should feel ashamed of and feeling shame that one is ashamed of feeling because one does not actually accept the standards on which it is based. Some of these things will be examined more fully later. I bring in this digression at this point in order that the aspects of shame described, in particular the feeling of inappropriateness and incongruity, may be seen as not necessarily wholly dependent on acceptance of the standards of the immediate society.

Finding oneself in a position of incongruity, not being accepted as the person one thought one was, not feeling at home in a world one thought one knew, can occur repeatedly throughout life. Sudden awareness of discrepancy may be brought about by changes in the social situation, for example, in a society of great mobility where an individual may unexpectedly find himself in an unfamiliar position, with the things he had taken for granted no longer there; or it may come about through changes in the person which put him out of key with a stable situation; or through changes outside the range of the more visible social structure.[b]

The loss of the identity one thought one had is in many ways more painful and disconcerting than the tortuous process of discovering identity that Shaw describes. This feeling of loss of identity can come about through changes in relations to one's family or friends or through changes in a professional or social situation to which one was committed. It is one of the painful characteristics of old age. The very identifications of oneself with one's body, one's mind, and the responses of other persons to the person one has been are no longer there and cannot be relied upon. Awareness of these changes in identity as they occur may be a special anguish.

> How can it really be
> That I was that young Tess
> And that before long I shall be
> The 'old princess,' the old wife of the Field Marshal?
> Look! There goes the old Duchess Theresia.
> How can it happen?
> Why should God do it
> While I am I and remain I?
> And if He does it
> Why does He permit me
> To look at all this with so clear a mind? [a]

The disconcertion arising from this juxtaposition of different perspectives explains the Biblical association of shame with confusion and confounding.* One is confounded by the inappropriate, and at a loss as to the means of restoring congruity.

Lear felt shame over the uncontrollable tears which were inappropriate for a king and for a man:

> Life and death! I am asham'd
> That thou hast power to shake my manhood thus;
> That these hot tears, which break from me perforce,
> Should make thee worth them. . . .[b]

Rejected by his daughters so that he felt himself

> . . . [a] slave,
> A poor, infirm, weak, and despis'd old man[c]

he struggled to regain his sense of congruence by proclaiming himself "every inch a king!" [d]

Dostoevski sensed with peculiar sensitivity congruence and incongruence and the lasting impact of the exposure involved in "unseemly" or inappropriate behavior. [e]

* It is this disconcertion that is the basis of the aspect of shame called embarrassment. Webster defines embarrass as: to hinder from liberty of thought or movement, to impede, perplex, or disconcert. Embarrassment is often an initial feeling in shame before shame is either covered up or explored as a means of further understanding of oneself and of the situation that gave rise to it.

. . . fifteen years later I should still in my imagination see Liza, always with the pitiful, distorted, inappropriate smile which was on her face at that minute.[a]

Virginia Woolf liked to think of herself as indifferent to public opinion, striving in her writing only to find the best artistic medium for her perceptions. The discovery that the appraisals of reviewers could wound her violated in disconcerting fashion her image of herself.

. . . opened the *Spectator* and read W. L. on me again. . . . Well L. says I should be contemptible to mind. Yes: but I do mind for 10 minutes: I mind being in the light again. . . . I must take a pull on myself. . . . I think I shall be free from the infection by Monday.[b]

Tolstoy makes clear both the shame of discrepancy arising from the sudden loss of all known landmarks in oneself and in the world, and the way in which one seizes upon familiar details of daily life in an effort to regain a sense of one's own identity and rootedness in the social situation.

Of Anna Karenina, surprised in the shameful awareness of her feeling for Vronsky as she journeyed from Moscow to Petersburg, he says:

. . . something seemed to choke her, and all objects and sounds in the wavering semi-darkness surprised her by their exaggerated proportions. She kept having moments of doubt as to whether the train were going backwards or forwards, or were standing still altogether; was it Annuska there, sitting next her, or was it a stranger?

"What is that on the hook?—my fur shuba or an animal? And what am I doing here? Am I myself, or some one else?" [c]

When Anna reached home she immersed herself in the familiar to dispel shame.

The hour before dinner . . . she employed sitting with her son . . . in arranging her things, and in reading and answering the letters and notes heaped up on her writing-table.

The sensation of causeless shame, and the agitation from which she had suffered so strangely during her journey, now completely disappeared. Under the conditions of her ordinary every-day life, she felt calm, and free from reproach, and she was filled with wonder as she recalled her condition of the night before.[a]

Different as Levin was from Anna, his experience of the shame of incongruity and of the surmounting of shame paralleled hers.

On the journey he . . . was overcome by the chaos of conflicting opinions, self-dissatisfaction, and a sense of shame. But when he got out at his station, and perceived his one-eyed coachman, Ignat, with his Kaftan collar turned up; . . . when Ignat, as he was tucking in the robes, told him all the news of the village . . . then it seemed to him that the chaos resolved itself a little, and his shame and dissatisfaction passed away. . . .

He felt himself again, and no longer wished to be a different person.[b]

It is peculiarly characteristic of these situations of suddenly experienced incongruity or discrepancy that evoke shame that they are often occasioned by what seems a "ridiculously" slight incident. An ostensibly trivial incident has precipitated intense emotion. What has occurred is harmless in itself and has no evil pragmatic outcome. It is the very triviality of the cause—an awkward gesture, a gaucherie in dress or table manners, "an untimely joke" always "a source of bitter regret,"[c] a gift or a witticism that falls flat, an expressed naïveté in taste, a mispronounced word, ignorance of some unimportant detail that everyone else surprisingly knows—that helps to give shame its unbearable character. "Some of those eccentricities are less often pardoned than vices," says Balzac of Père Goriot.[d] "Men blush for their crimes much less than for their weaknesses or vanity."[e] "Goldsmith was reserved because his foibles are of the kind men conceal; his ludicrous mishaps in dress, his preoccupation with his ugliness and awkwardness, his poverty, his fear of ridicule."[f]

Tolstoy makes the fact that shame is an open wound occasioned by a slight incident one of the distinctions between shame and guilt. He says of Levin:

There had been in his past, as in every man's, actions recognized by him as bad, for which his conscience ought to have tormented him; but the memory of these evil actions was far from causing him so much suffering as these trivial but humiliating reminiscences. These wounds never healed.[a]

Part of Dostoevski's power lies in his revelation of the way in which an outwardly trivial incident can become invested with profound human emotion and be transformed into an event of tremendous import. It was this slight occasion for much feeling that bewildered Velchaninov.

. . . he felt as though someone had caught him in something shameful. He was bewildered and surprised.

"Then there must be reasons for my being so angry . . . apropos of nothing . . . at a mere reminiscence." [b]

It is in part because of his realization of the informing power for the individual of the seemingly insignificant that Dostoevski's novels, whatever his intentions, can never be primarily political or religious tracts, nor any of his characters simply an embodiment of an idea. Stavrogin's attention could always remain held by "a trifle." Mary Lebyatkin could blush and become "terribly ashamed" over a "slight accident" as she did not over her position as the unacknowledged wife of Stavrogin —or rather the fall could suddenly bring her bodily awkwardness and her whole position into painful awareness; Mrs. Stavrogin's calling the Sistine Madonna the Dresden Madonna could bring into focus the whole of her relation to Mrs. Lembke.[c] It is for this reason, too, that no matter how sordid the details that Dostoevski introduces they never remain only sordid, and that it is difficult for him to remain wholly alien from any of his characters. He *is* the four brothers Karamazov; he is Mr. Verkhovensky as well as Shatov and Kirilov; General Yepanchin as well as Myshkin.[d]

Faulkner's *Light in August* is a study in shame. Here, too, it is the small details that probe the depths of pain. More than in his uncertainty about his Negro blood, more than in the indignity of McEachern's cruelty or his wife's self-distrustful kindness, Christmas feels shame in the details of his relation with Bobby, the waitress—the discovery that pie and coffee cost fifteen cents instead of the dime he had, his return to repay the extra nickel, his ignorance about "woman's sickness" and of "what one does" in the sex act, his first gift to Bobby of the stale and fly-specked box of candy. The newness and uniqueness of his gift was as important as the newness and uniqueness he felt in her body. After his discovery that she was a prostitute he had to regain his position *with himself* by repudiating his own shyness, decency, and tenderness.[a]

Because of the outwardly small occasion that has precipitated shame, the intense emotion seems inappropriate, incongruous, disproportionate to the incident that has aroused it. Hence a double shame is involved; we are ashamed because of the original episode and ashamed because we feel so deeply about something so slight that a sensible person would not pay any attention to it. "We no more forgive an emotion for showing itself completely than we forgive a man for not having a cent," says Balzac.[b]

Various interpretations can be made of the fact that a seemingly trivial occurrence can give rise to feelings of intense shame. Some people would regard feeling acute shame over a slight gaucherie as neurotic.[c] Others think that trivial shame and neurotic shame should be placed in separate categories distinct from real shame and existentialist shame.[d] I believe that both of these interpretations miss the importance of the way in which a trifling incident can touch off a deep sense of shame. It is true that a consistent and excessive response of shame over using the wrong fork or mispronouncing a word may in some cases be a sign of neurotic or even psychotic tendencies. It is also true that a trivial incident will presumably produce less shame in a situation and with persons where one feels relatively secure and at home. But to assume that any feeling of deep shame over a seemingly trivial incident is neurotic is to miss the point that it is characteristic of shame, as experienced by normal, healthy persons, that a seemingly insignificant occurrence can set off a train of associations that have profound significance for the whole self.* Freud made this

* For precisely this effect of a trivial incident see the discussion of Virginia Woolf's "The New Dress," p. 53. The normality of the character pictured there may be questioned, but not, I think, the normal nature of the experience.

very clear in the *Psychopathology of Everyday Life.*[a] It is also the case that the very fact of feeling at home in a situation and then suddenly discovering that it is alien can be disconcertingly touched off by a slight occurrence.

One other point should be mentioned in connection with shame as sudden awareness of discrepancy. The same situation of suddenly exposed incongruity can give rise to shame or to laughter. Different explanations of this fact according to different theories of personality will be discussed later.

Threat to Trust

In an experience of shame trust is seriously jeopardized or destroyed. Emphasis may fall on one side or the other: on the questioning of one's own adequacy or on the questioning of the values in the world of reality which so contradict what one has been led to expect. Or both may be doubted. In any case, suddenly exposed discrepancy threatens trust. Part of the difficulty in admitting shame to oneself arises from reluctance to recognize that one has built on false assumptions about what the world one lives in is and about the way others will respond to oneself There is a failure to meet on common ground, as, for example, when adolescent children suddenly find their parents strangers, or when one meets a trusted friend after a separation and finds that the years have taken each person in a different direction.

Shame over a sudden uncovering of incongruity mounts when what is exposed is inappropriate positive expectation, happy and confident commitment to a world that proves to be alien or nonexistent.

> They are confused because of their trust;
> They come to the spot and are put to shame.[b]

Even more than the uncovering of weakness or ineptness, exposure of misplaced confidence can be shameful—happiness, love, anticipation of a response that is not there, something personally momentous received as inconsequential.* The greater the expectation, the more acute the shame; the greater the discrepancy between one's image of oneself and the image others have of one, the more one has to "put on a brave face."

The gift-giving of a child to an older person whose orientation is different offers special occasions for such shame. A child spent a whole morning and infinite care constructing a necklace of paper discs and links as a surprise gift for an old lady who was to be an afternoon guest. With the construction went the blissful anticipation of the delight of the recipient, and debate as to the best way to present the gift. She finally decided that the surprise and pleasure would be greater if she slipped the necklace over the head of the guest. The years of a lifetime would not be enough to erase the shame aroused by the guest's impatient response. "Take this thing off my head, Jenny, it's tearing my hair net."

A small girl pictured the delight of her older brother when she presented him with a jigsaw puzzle of a mountain scene, found after much search, and paid for out of her allowance—but he had outgrown puzzles. "Do you still like detective stories?" she asked eagerly, producing a pocket Sherlock Holmes—but he was reading Malraux. Similar violation of expectation occurs if an adult treats casually or indifferently an event such as a school or Scout ceremony of momentous importance to a child.

Not only children experience the confusion resulting from such blocking of a vital act of special importance, or such careless dismissal of a value-loaded gift. A mother may offer to her daughter a set of china or fine damask, the treasure of a lifetime, as a supreme gesture of devotion—to be met with an open or disguised response that this is unwanted, old-fashioned junk.

Aldous Huxley's despair of human beings arises in part from his belief that any expectation of positive response from other persons inevitably ends in humiliation.

* Harry Stack Sullivan has described this collapse of a bedrock relation. See pp. 151, 156, 162-3, 212-3 for discussion of Sullivan's views.

At the sound of that telephone voice Elinor quickly drew away from him. To press yourself against someone who turns out simply not to be there is not only disappointing; it is also rather humiliating. Which evenings, indeed! [a]

In a very different mood Turgenev describes expectation unrealized. The aging composer Lemm thought he had for once captured his dreams in a song composed to express his love and admiration for Lisa.

> . . . Lisa sat down . . . to the piano and played . . . the song. . . . Alas! the music turned out to be complicated and painfully strained; it was clear that the composer had striven to express something passionate and deep, but nothing had come of it; the effort had remained an effort. Lavretsky and Lisa both felt this, and Lemm understood it. Without uttering a single word, he put his song back into his pocket, and in reply to Lisa's proposal to play it again, he only shook his head and said significantly: 'Now—enough!' and *shrinking into himself* he turned away.[b] (Italics mine.)

Basic trust in the personal and in the physical world that surrounds him is the air that the child must breathe if he is to have roots for his own sense of identity and for the related sense of his place in the world. As he gradually differentiates the world of in here from the world of out there he is constantly testing the coherence, continuity, and dependability of both.[c] Things that for an adult have defined outlines and constancies for a child remain fluid and must slowly coalesce. Schachtel beautifully describes the way in which a child's insistence on the word-for-word repetition of a familiar story is a demand for assurance that it is *there*,[d] to be depended upon; alteration may be as disconcerting for him as it would be for an adult to see a familiar house or mountain suddenly standing on its apex. The developing sense of himself and the developing sense of the world about him increase concurrently.* Expectation and having expectation met are crucial in developing a sense of coherence in the world and in oneself.

* See n. 138c for a questioning of this view.

Sudden experience of a violation of expectation, of incongruity between expectation and outcome, results in a shattering of trust in oneself, even in one's own body and skill and identity, and in the trusted boundaries or framework of the society and the world one has known. As trust in oneself and in the outer world develop together, so doubt of oneself and of the world are also intermeshed.

The rejected gift, the joke or the phrase that does not come off, the misunderstood gesture, the falling short of our own ideals, the expectation of response violated—such experiences mean that we have trusted ourselves to a situation that is not there. We have relied on the assumption of one perspective or *Gestalt* and found a totally different one. What we have thought we could count on in ourselves, and what we have thought to be the boundaries and contours of the world, turn out suddenly not to be the "real" outlines of ourselves or of the world, or those that others accept. We have become strangers in a world where we thought we were at home. We experience anxiety in becoming aware that we cannot trust our answers to the questions Who am I? Where do I belong?

A child taken abroad at four had just begun to become accustomed to the strangeness of life on shipboard when there began to be talk of landing in a strange country, of going to a strange hotel. She protested, "I don't want to go there. Nobody will know me."

Few people have realized as deeply as George Eliot the irreplaceable character of trusted early surroundings. She describes

> . . . that familiar hearth, where the pattern of the rug, and the grate, and the fire irons were "first ideas" that it was no more possible to criticize than the solidity and extension of matter.
>
> . . . There is no sense of ease like the ease we felt in those scenes where we were born, where objects became dear to us before we had known the labor of choice, and where the outer world seemed only an extension of our own personality: we accepted and loved it as we accepted our own sense of existence and our own limbs.[a]

Because personality is rooted in unconscious and unquestioned trust in one's immediate world, experiences that shake trusted anticipations and give rise to doubt may be of lasting importance. In Elizabethan English doubt and fear were synonymous. "Do not doubt that," says Desdemona,[a] meaning "Trust; do not fear." Doubt replacing basic trust in the way of life of one's social group or in one's place in it can undermine the sense of one's own identity. Thus shame, an experience of violation of trust in oneself and in the world, may go deeper than guilt for a specific act. The emphasis on strict moral codes and hatred of sin which characterize certain cultures and certain periods of history may actually arise from a basic distrust of life.

Shattering of trust in the dependability of one's immediate world means loss of trust in other persons, who are the transmitters and interpreters of that world. We have relied on the picture of the world they have given us and it has proved mistaken; we have turned for response in what we thought was a relation of mutuality and have found our expectation misinterpreted or distorted; we have opened ourselves in anticipation of a response that was not forthcoming. With every recurrent violation of trust we become again children unsure of ourselves in an alien world.

An old volume, little known now, gives an exceptionally sensitive account of a child trustingly and earnestly trying to find her way in the bewildering adult world of arbitrary signs.

> It was when a bell rang one must stand up. But what for, Emmy Lou never knew, until after the others began to do it.
>
> . . . to be told crossly to sit down was bewildering, when in answer to c, a, t, one said "Pussy." And yet there was Pussy washing her face on the chart, and Miss Clara's pointer pointing to her.[b]
> . . . the music man drew . . . five lines on the blackboard, and made eight dots. . . . "This," said Mr. Cato, "is A," and he pointed to a dot. . . . "A," said Emmy Lou, obediently . . . she had met A in so many guises of print and script that she accepted any statement concerning A. And now a dot was A.
>
> ". . . but we are not going to call them A, B, C, D, E, F, G, A [said Mr. Cato] . . . we are going to call them do, re, mi, fa, sol, la, si. . . . A is do here. Always remember the first letter in the scale is do."
>
> . . . [In spelling class] the rest might forget, but Emmy Lou would not. It came her turn.

She stood up. Her word was Adam. And A was dough. Emmy Lou went slowly to get it right. "Dough-d-dough-m, Adam," said Emmy Lou.

They laughed.[a]

Norbert Wiener describes the bewilderment of a child when trusted interpretations of his world fail him:

Christmas of 1901 was hard for me. I was just seven. It was then that I first discovered that Santa Claus was a conventional invention of the grownups. At that time I was already reading scientific books of more than slight difficulty, and it seemed to my parents that a child who was doing this should have no difficulty in discarding what to them was obviously a sentimental fiction. What they did not realize was the fragmentariness of the child's world. The child does not wander far from home, and what may be only a few blocks away is to him an unknown territory in which every fancy is permissible.

What is true concerning the physical map is also true concerning the chart of his ideas. He has not yet had the opportunity to explore very far from the few central notions that are his by experience. In the intermediate regions, anything may be true; and what for his elders is at least an emotional contradiction is for him a blank which may be filled in any one of several ways.[b]

The discovery that our parents are not all-wise and all-good and that we must face the uncertainties of our own judgment and our own interpretations of the world is a lonely experience. It becomes still more lonely and poignant, and in a real sense shameful, when it is followed by the realization that, instead of our elders being our interpreters of the world, our protectors, we must, instead, protect them from their own fallibilities and shortcomings, and from the shameful knowledge that we are aware of them.

This painful transformation of roles appears in Rilke's account of the metamorphosis of birthdays.

. . . on [one's birthday] one arose with a right to joy which was not to be doubted. . . .

But suddenly come those remarkable birthdays when . . . you see others becoming uncertain. . . . You are hardly awake when someone shouts . . . that the cake hasn't arrived yet; . . . or somebody comes in and leaves the door open, and you see everything before you should have seen it. That is the moment when something like an operation is performed on you: a brief but atrociously painful incision. . . . You have scarce got over it when you no longer think about yourself; you must rescue the birthday, watch the others, anticipate their mistakes, and confirm them in the illusion that they are managing everything admirably. . . . They want to surprise you and . . . [they] open the lowest layer of a toy-box which contains nothing more, only cotton-wool; then you have to relieve their embarrassment.[a]

To some extent everyone experiences a loss of early trust,[b] which may leave a nostalgia for familiar images unmarred by change. But the extent to which some form of early trust continues for a person, and the way in which it is transmuted into more mature and understanding confidence, determine in important ways his future sense of identity.

Involvement of the Whole Self

Shame is an experience that affects and is affected by the whole self. This whole-self involvement is one of its distinguishing characteristics and one that makes it a clue to identity.

Separate, discrete acts or incidents, including those seemingly most trivial, have importance because in this moment of *self*-consciousness, the self stands revealed. Coming suddenly upon us, experiences of shame throw a flooding light on what and who we are and what the world we live in is.

This gives at least a partial answer to the question as to whether shame is something that one voluntarily brings on oneself or something that comes upon one from without. It is both. One does not, as in guilt, choose to engage in a specific act, a sin. Guilt frequently involves a sort of haggling anxiety, a weighing of pros and cons prolonged over a period of time. The shameful situation frequently takes one by surprise. But one is overtaken by shame because one's whole life has been a preparation for putting one in this situation. One finds oneself in a situation in which hopes and purposes are invested and in which anxiety about one's own adequacy may also be felt. In shame the inadequacy becomes manifest; the anxiety is realized. It is because of this whole-life involvement that one can speak of an over-all ashamedness. Jean-Paul Sartre makes basic in shame the way one appears in the eyes of others (others as audience), rather than in one's own eyes. But he recognizes that what is exposed in shame is oneself. I am ashamed of what I am.[a]

Because of this over-all character, an experience of shame can be altered or transcended only in so far as there is some change in the whole self.[b] No single, specific thing we can do can rectify or mitigate such an experience. Unlike guilt it is—in specific terms—irreversible. "In shame there is no comfort, but to be beyond all bounds of shame." It is too small to refer to; but it pervades everything. There it is. An experience that arouses guilt, from a slight misdemeanor to a crime, can be followed by appropriate mitigating or nullifying sequences—confession, repentance, punishment, atonement, condemnation, restoration. "Even the misery of guilt doth attain to the bliss of pardon." At least in our culture, guilt is a culturally defined wrong act, a part of oneself that is separable, segmented, and redeemable.

But an experience of shame of the sort I am attempting to describe cannot be modified by addition, or wiped out by subtraction, or exorcised by expiation.[c] It is not an isolated act that can be detached from the self. It carries the weight of "I cannot have done this. But I have done it and I cannot undo it, because this is I." It is pervasive as anxiety is pervasive;[d] its focus is not a separate act, but revelation of the whole self. The thing that has been exposed is what I am.

To describe these experiences as loss of face or acting in an unsuitable role is inadequate, because these formulations are relatively external. The German language, as noted earlier, reflects the direction of the quality of shame, inseparable from the depths of the self, in contrast to guilt, as it reflects the similar distinction between anxiety and fear: *Ich schäme mich,* but *Ich bin schuldig; Ich ängste mich,* but *Ich fürchte etwas.* Guilt can be expiated. Shame, short of a transformation of the self, is retained. This transformation means, in Plato's words, a turning of the whole soul toward the light.

Piers' distinction between shame and guilt, quoted above, is rooted in the shattering of one's sense of self in shame, in the failure to reach one's ideal:*

> Whereas guilt is generated whenever a boundary . . . is touched or transgressed, shame occurs when a goal . . . is not being reached. It thus indicates a real "short-coming." Guilt anxiety accompanies transgression; shame, failure.
>
> . . . the Ego-Ideal is in continuous dynamic interfunction with the unconscious and conscious *awareness of the Ego's potentialities.*
>
> Shame . . . occurs whenever goals and images presented by the Ego-Ideal are not reached.[a]

With all the emphasis on codified guilt that is part of our Western heritage, there is abundant evidence in our literature of recognition of the distinction between specific acts that are, in a sense, detachable from the self because they may be punished or expiated and those acts and feelings that reveal the whole person. Alcibiades says of his feeling in the presence of Socrates:

> When I hear him my heart leaps in me more than that of the Corybantes; my tears flow at his words. . . . And with this man alone I have an experience which no one would believe was possible for me—the sense of shame. . . . Often I would be glad if I should not see him again in this world, but if this should happen I know very well that I should be more miserable than ever. . . .[b]

Othello makes clear the difference between shame in the Freud-Benedict sense of reaction to the ridicule of others,

> . . . to make me
> A fixed figure for the time of scorn
> To point his slow unmoving finger at![c]

and the far deeper, more unbearable wound which cuts to the center of the self,

* See pp. 166-71 for discussion of the relation between the self or ego, the self-image, and the ego ideal.

> . . . there where I have garner'd up my heart,
> Where either I must live or bear no life,
> The fountain from the which my current runs
> Or else dries up. . . .[a]

This cry of Othello's also points again to the relation between being overtaken by a situation of shame and a voluntary act of choice. The circumstances of Desdemona's supposed betrayal came upon Othello; the situation was not the result of an immediate act of choice. But he was in this situation because he was the kind of person he was, a person who had chosen Desdemona and chosen Iago.

This feeling of a crumpling or failure of the whole self appears in Dmitri Furmanov's description of his hero Klychkov, who has experienced cowardice in his first hours under fire.

> Oh! Shame, unspeakable, unutterable shame! It was bitter to realize that his heart had failed him in the first battle, that he had fallen short of his own expectations. Where had been the boldness, the heroism of which he had dreamed so much when he was still far from the front line? [b]

A similar sense of shame at failure to be what one thought one was, although no one else was aware of the incident, appears in a recent American volume of science fiction. The seventeen-year-old hero sees a Negro boy pursued by a man on horseback with the clear intent of riding him down. He did not hold on to the rein and delay the hunter:

> I had been immobilized by the fear of asserting my sympathies, my presumptions, against events.
>
> . . . Walking slowly down the road I experienced deep shame. I might, I could have saved someone from hurt; I had perhaps had the power for a brief instant to change the course of a whole life.
>
> . . . I couldn't excuse my failure on the grounds that action would have been considered outrageous. It would not have been considered outrageous by me.[c]

Samuel Stouffer describing the common experience of fear in battle—often known only to oneself—makes it clear that this failure to live up to one's expectations of oneself is related not to one particular aspect of personality but to a whole cluster of ideals.*

Conceptions of masculinity vary among different American groups, but there is a core which is common to most: courage, endurance and toughness, lack of squeamishness . . . avoidance of display of weakness in general, reticence about emotional or idealistic matters, and sexual competency. . . .

A code as universal as "being a man" is very likely to have been deeply internalized. So the fear of failure in the role, as by showing cowardice in battle, could bring not only fear of social censure on this point as such, but also more central and strongly established fears related to sex-typing:

. . . behavior in combat was recognized as a test of being a man . . . a man once in combat had to fight in order to keep his own self-respect: "Hell, I'm a soldier." [a]

In "The New Dress" Virginia Woolf shows how one incident takes on an unbearably wounding character because this single occasion partakes of and reveals what one's whole life has been and is. It was not only that Mabel's new yellow dress, so carefully contrived with the little dressmaker, stood out at Mrs. Dalloway's party as conspicuous, ridiculous, "not *right.*" Since it was not right, it made Mabel question her feeling for Miss Milan, who had made it, and her own earlier happiness in the making of it; it made her question her "safe" marriage to Hubert, her "fretful, weak, unsatisfactory" motherhood, her "wobbly" feeling as a wife; her own appalling inadequacy; her cowardice; her "mean, water-sprinkled blood." [b]

Because of the pervasive and specifically unalterable character of experiences of shame, shame for one's parents can pierce deeper than shame for oneself, and sense of continuity with one's parents is correspondingly important. No matter how dis-

* Grinker and Spiegel say that men who leave combat because of overpowering anxiety are haunted by depression over failure to live up to their own and the group's standards of courageous performance. The effect of military service is, not only to create resentment of discipline and of curtailment of personal interest, but even more to lead to the incorporation of military demands into the personality of the soldier. (Roy R. Grinker and John P. Spiegel, *Men Under Stress,* Blakiston, 1945, pp. 40, 114, 279.)

gusted I am with myself, in some respects I can perhaps change. But the fact that these are my parents, that I am the fruit of their loins, is unchangeable. "Shame in a kindred cannot be avoided," says a seventeenth-century proverb.

Myth and literature recognize the special character of shame felt by children for their parents. Noah's sons felt this shame when

> Noah . . . drank of the wine, and was drunken; and he was uncovered within his tent. . . . And Shem and Japheth took a garment, and laid it upon both their shoulders, and went backward, and covered the nakedness of their father; and their faces were backward, and they saw not their father's nakedness.[a]

Albany, upbraiding Goneril for her treatment of her father, says

> That nature which contemns its origin
> Cannot be bordered certain in itself.
> She that herself will sliver and disbranch
> From her material sap, perforce must wither
> And come to deadly use.[b]

Pierre's whole life and self were uprooted when he discovered that he had all his life been cherishing a false image of the integrity of his father.

> He looked up, and found himself fronted by the no longer wholly enigmatical, but still ambiguously smiling picture of his father . . . endure the smiling portrait he could not; and obeying an irresistible nameless impulse, he rose, and without unhanging it, reversed the picture on the wall.[c]

The Brothers Karamazov is a delineation of the varieties of shame that bound each son to his father. Elsewhere Dostoevski explores the same theme.

> Velchaninov . . . guessed that [Liza] was ashamed before *him,* that she was ashamed of her father's having so easily let her go with him, of his having, as it were, flung her into his keeping.[d]

Flora de Barral felt such shame for her father:

> The girl was like a creature struggling under a net. "But how can I forget she called my father a cheat and a swindler? It can't be true. How can it be true?"

> . . . Flora . . . who *felt the shame but did not believe in the guilt* of her father, retorted fiercely: "Nevertheless, I am as honourable as you are." [a] (Italics mine.)

The enormous perceptiveness of children in sensing unease or hypocrisy in their parents and their shame when they are aware that their parents are acting a part appears in *Anna Karenina:*

> The little girl well knew that there was trouble between her father and her mother, and that her mother could not be cheerful, and that her father ought to know it, and that he was dissembling when he questioned her so lightly. And she blushed for her father.[b]

Elizabeth Bennet "blushed and blushed again with shame and vexation" at her mother's improprieties at the Netherfield ball, but, because of her greater closeness to her father, felt an even deeper pang at his complacency when it seemed to her that "her family [had] made an agreement to expose themselves." [c]

For Virginia Woolf it was a terrible experience, when her father made a scene, to have to excuse him for being "so majestic and so unreasonable." "It was also belittling to his real dignity that they knew he would be sorry later on and would reproach himself bitterly and need to be comforted because he was such an unkind father." [d] Of the description of her father as Mr. Ramsay in *To the Lighthouse* Virginia Woolf said, "I am more like him than [my mother] and therefore more critical." [e]

For a child of immigrant parents there is often acute conflict between the desire to look up to his parents and the shame he feels for the exposure of their different ways and their uncertainty and unseemliness in a strange land.[f] Estranged from both cultures he may manifest his own insecurity about where he belongs by overzealousness in taking on the ways of the school and the neighborhood alien to his elders, and by impatience with their foreignness and slowness of adaptation.

Less extreme than the predicament of the child of immigrant parents is the widely felt, if not widely acknowledged, shame of children who become aware that their parents are not secure or at home in their social environment. This may occur with parents of modest financial means who are ill at ease with or accept favors from those who have more; or with parents who are gentle in a society that demands efficiency, or who place other values before achievement and success but show diffidence in doing so. Deference toward other persons on the part of parents, their not "knowing what to do" in a situation that calls for competence, their smiling acquiescence in place of strength, may arouse in their children pity or protectiveness when they want to give respect—a feeling hard to acknowledge and hard to bear.

Such feeling toward one's parents may be in varying degrees a more common human experience than we realize. The over-all quality of shame involves the whole life of a person, all that he is, including the parents who have created and nurtured that life.

Confronting of Tragedy

The import of shame for others may reach even deeper than shame for ourselves.[a] This is true not only of shame for our parents, but in very different ways of feeling shame with other persons less close to us, and, in still different ways, of feeling shame for and with our children.

Identifications with other persons in situations that make them feel ashamed lead beyond such experiences of shame as have been described to the confrontation of the human condition and the possibilities and the tragic limitations of man's lot. This confrontation may be the beginning of the realization of shame as revelation—of oneself, of one's society, and of the world—and of the transcending of shame.

Loss of trust, exposure, failure, the feeling of homelessness—these experiences of shame—become still more unbearable if they lead to the feeling that there is no home for anyone, anywhere. Paradoxically, shame, an isolating, highly personal experience is also peculiarly related to one's conception of the universe, and of one's place in it. Apprehension that one's own life may be cut off from others, empty, void of significance, is a terrifying thing; but fear that this same isolation is true for others, and that the world itself may hold no meaning is infinitely worse. Experience of shame may call into question, not only one's own adequacy and the validity of the codes of one's immediate society, but the meaning of the universe itself.

It is one thing to recognize the inevitable limitations of man's lot—that even the longest life of man is no more than a hundred years and ends in death; that death separates us from those we love; that in a single life we can realize only a few of the possibilities within us for creative work and love; that in imagination we can go backward and forward in time and space but are actually alive in only limited parts of the world and in only one age. It is a wholly different thing to say that life is nothing but tragedy, that life holds, or can discover, no meaning except that it leads toward death. We may not be able to affirm with St. Augustine that

> He who knows the Truth knows that [Unchangeable] Light; and he that knows it knoweth eternity. . . . I should more readily doubt that I live than that Truth [exists]. . . . For that truly is which remains immutably.[a]

But the demand to discover or to create significance in life asserts itself no less insistently. There are times when we feel that more than anything else in the world we should like to have—for just a few moments—the perspective of a God's-eye view of situations in which we are involved. Depending on initial premises, we can sort experiences this way or that with logic and validity. But what is the True, the Right, way to sort them? "I want to be there when every one suddenly understands what it has all been for," says Ivan Karamazov.

Feeling with others in situations of exposure, estrangement, forces us to face the questions of whether there is meaning and where truth and meaning lie. Lionel Trilling in his story "The Other Margaret" beautifully describes the way in which shame for another may lead to a questioning of meaning in life. Such questions come to the fore when we feel shame for and with others in circumstances from the most humble to the most august.

The child depicted in *Emmy Lou* painfully, if dimly, felt these questions through seeing the humiliation of Lisa Schmit, the daughter of a German grocer.

> One day the air of the Fourth Reader room . . . was most unpleasant.
>
> "Who in this room has lunch?" said Miss Lizzie. . . . "File by the platform in order, bringing your lunch" . . . Some were in newspaper. Emmy Lou's heart ached for those. . . . Miss Lizzie bent and deliberately smelled of each package in turn. . . . Most of the faces of the little girls were red.
>
> Then came Lisa—Lisa Schmit. Her lunch was in paper—heavy brown paper. . . .
>
> "Open it," said Miss Lizzie.
>
> . . . The unpleasantness wafted heavily. There was sausage and dark gray bread and cheese. It was the cheese that was unpleasant.
>
> "Go open the stove door," said Miss Lizzie. "Now, take it and put it in. . . ."
>
> Lisa took her lunch and put it in. . . . When she got back to her seat, Lisa's head went down on her arm on the desk, and . . . even her yellow plaits shook with the convulsiveness of her sobs.
>
> It wasn't the loss of the sausage or the bread or the cheese, Emmy Lou . . . knew.[a]

Acknowledgment of personal sin or confession of guilt may sometimes be a defense against the possibility that there may be no meaning in the world. After some experiences of shame and fear of emptiness we may welcome guilt as a friend. Sin, guilt, punishment—each is, in one sense, an affirmation of order and significance. Shame questions the reality of any significance. Guilt in oneself is easier to face than lack of meaning in life.

Philip, praying with utter faith that his clubfoot would be made whole, found it better to believe that he lacked faith than that God had failed him.

> "D'you mean to say [said Philip] that if you really believed you could move mountains you could?"
>
> "By the grace of God," said the Vicar.

. . . he . . . prayed to God with all his might that He would make his club-foot whole. It was a very small thing beside the moving of mountains. . . .

"Oh, God, . . . if it be Thy will, please make my foot all right on the night before I go back to school."

. . . No doubts assailed him. He was confident in the word of God . . . the morning for the miracle. . . . His first instinct was to put down his hand and feel the foot which was whole now, but to do this seemed to doubt the goodness of God. He knew that his foot was well. But at last he made up his mind, and with the toes of his right foot he just touched his left. Then he passed his hand over it. . . .

. . . perhaps he had not given God enough time. . . . But presently the feeling came to him that this time also his faith would not be great enough.

"I suppose no one ever has faith enough," he said.[a]

George Eliot's Dorothea in Rome showed a similar eagerness to exaggerate her own guilt rather than to admit inadequacy in the possibilities of love or loss of faith in the people and the world she had trusted. However just her indignation might be, "her ideal was not to claim justice, but to give tenderness."[b] So, too, Anna Karenina would go to any length in order not to recognize that the love between her and Vronsky was less than she had believed.

Having read the letter, [Vronsky] raised his eyes to her, and there was no determination in them. . . . She knew that whatever he might say to her, he would not say all he thought. And she knew that her last hope had failed. . . .

"You say degrading . . . don't say that . . ." she said in a shaking voice. She did not want him now to say what was untrue. Her love for him was trembling in the balance. . . . "If [your love] is like mine, I feel so exalted, so strong, that nothing can be humiliating to me. I am proud of my position, because . . ." She could not say what she was proud of. Tears of shame and despair choked her utterance.[c]

Shame for one's children raises other searching questions. Just as shame for and with one's parents in some ways tests the limits of one's acceptance of oneself, so shame for and with one's children—their feelings of inferiority and failure, their disappointment in positive expectations of other people and of the world—comes near to testing the limits of one's faith in the possibilities of life. The sensitivity of this area of awareness is suggested by the fact that many people would hesitate to speak of shame for their children. If the feeling of shame for one's children receives psychological recognition it is quickly codified as a parental defect.

At least two things obscure recognition of some of the implications of identifications with our children which partake of the nature of shame.

The first takes the more obvious forms of desiring the success of our children in terms of the standards of the culture or of our particular group in the culture ("intellectuals" may repudiate the cruder and more common success norms and set up their own even more exigent ones) and of feeling some sort of shame for our children if these are not attained. This is a phenomenon widely recognized and discussed as a characteristic of American life.[a] Many of us do, more than we like to admit, want, among other values, such success for our children. It is undeniably true that many parents do want to realize themselves through pride in their children's achievements, to have their children succeed where they themselves have fallen short. But if we stop here we have barely touched the edge of what identifications with one's children imply.

A second factor that confuses entering into the deeper implications of these identifications is that the complex of feelings about our children's lives and hopes is one in which shame and guilt are peculiarly intermeshed. Consciousness of guilt and of where we have failed our children almost inevitably submerges awareness of the implications of shame. Few parents, as they watch the disappointments and frustrations, or the compromises and adjustments, of their children as they make their own choices in becoming related to social "reality" can escape some feeling that had they done certain things differently the path for their children might have been clearer.

Some of the social changes of the last quarter or half century have made growing up more difficult; and certain kinds of awareness of the way in which seemingly incidental aspects of behavior of parents may affect their children's lives* have heightened the parents' sense of responsibility and of wrongdoing.

Neither the obvious forms of what may be called shame if our children fall short of our wishes for their achievement nor the much more important guilt we feel over our own inadequacies toward them, however, come near to the core of the implications of our identifications with them. Something far deeper is involved in our desires for our children and the putting to trial through them of our faith in the possibilities of life. For ourselves we can accept disappointment, rebuff, and failure. Recognizing and accepting it for them becomes an almost wholly different experience.

> O my son Absalom, my son, my son Absalom!
> Would God I had died for thee,
> O Absalom, my son, my son!

The cry stands alone. The love and expectations of a father for his son, the guilt of a father for the way his son's life grew and ended, the treachery of a son toward his father[a]—it is beyond them all.

Is there anything in the world of adult reality that is commensurate with the uncertain excitement of a child in taking his first steps; the trust with which he holds out his arms to be taken up; his eager intensity as he digs in the sand, his laughter

* For the last twenty-five years or more, child psychologists have been warning parents, especially mothers, of all the things they must not do or be lest they permanently damage their children. Parents have been censured for being overstrict and overpermissive, overdetached and overprotective, and for a thousand other mistakes of commission and omission. In recent years, not altogether pleased at the results of these efforts, child psychologists have flown still another danger signal—parents must, at all costs, not be "overanxious parents"! The Mental Health Materials Center issues a pamphlet entitled "What Did I Do?" presenting "the case of a mother" who through trying too hard missed some important clues from her child. (Dorothy Barclay, "The Case of the Overanxious Parent," New York *Times Magazine*, May 5, 1957.)

Much recent work of child psychologists tries specifically to correct the effect of such guilt-producing injunctions.

as a wave breaks over him; the expectancy overcoming self-doubt with which an adolescent goes out to meet new people, new places, new ideas; the hope of an expanding world with which a freshman enters college; the wonder and dawning confidence of a first—and renewed—love?

Or, must we say that maturity involves the acceptance of frustrations of which earlier bewildered disappointments are prototypes: being excluded— "They're playing a game and I guess I'm not in it any more"; offering one's most cherished book, a much-read copy of *Treasure Island,* as a birthday present and having it disregarded among the new and costly gifts; the expectancy called forth by the words over a college entrance "The Pursuit of Truth" being met by rebuff and "scaling down to size"; open friendship met by formality; love by shrinking or betrayal?

And is the raising of such questions as these a mark of sentimentality and immaturity?

As shame of immigrant children for their parents highlights certain similar but less acute experiences of other children, so the feeling of these same parents for their children by its intensity illumines questions that present themselves in some form to many parents.

> About the children [the immigrant parents] can feel no certainty whatever.
>
> . . . It was difficult enough to show them the right ways around the corners of the city blocks; it was infinitely more difficult to show them the right ways around the twisting curves of the new way of life.
>
> . . . It occurs to [the parents] that they cannot possibly meet their obligations to the children . . . by the act of migration, they . . . have destroyed the birthright of their sons and daughters. . . . To each other, the parents acknowledge the guilt: *Yes, dear, and therefore let us sacrifice ourselves and live only for them. If there is any hope in this world, it is not for us but for them.*
>
> It was easier to bend the neck in readiness than to be certain that the yoke would fit. With bewilderment the immigrants learned that to be willing to sacrifice was not enough, that their children must

be also willing to accept the sacrifice; and of that there could be no confidence.[a]

For these parents, too, their children's future could become one test of their faith in life. "From the depths of a dark pessimism they looked up at a frustrating universe ruled by haphazard, capricious forces." [b] For them, too, the feeling of personal guilt was easier to bear than facing lack of meaning in the world.

Hardy describes Clym's bitter self-reproach as a refuge from facing lack of trust in other persons and ultimate emptiness.

He did sometimes think he had been ill-used by fortune, so far as to say that to be born is a palpable dilemma, and that instead of men aiming to advance in life with glory they should calculate how to retreat out of it without shame. But that he and his had been sarcastically and pitilessly handled in having such irons thrust into their souls he did not maintain long. It is usually so except with the sternest of men. Human beings, in their generous endeavour to construct a hypothesis that shall not degrade a First Cause, have always hesitated to conceive a dominant power of lower moral quality than their own; and, even while they sit down and weep by the waters of Babylon, invent excuses for the oppression which prompts their tears.[c]

Shame for God or for the world is harder to bear than shame for ourselves. We may think that Gloucester lacked courage or was without sense of historic change, but there are no more fearful words than his

> As flies to wanton boys are we to th' gods.
> They kill us for their sport.[d]

Failure to reach our own aspirations, our own possibilities, is intimately related to the way we see our place in the universe, and hence to the way we conceive the universe itself. This leads to the question of how far disappointment and the failure of human effort lie in the unalterable nature of things and how far in the particular version of the nature of things presented by our society and this period of history. This question, which presents itself repeatedly, will be discussed further.

Difficulty in Communicating Shame

The characteristics that have been suggested as central in experiences of shame—the sudden exposure of unanticipated incongruity, the seemingly trivial incident that arouses overwhelming and almost unbearably painful emotion, the threat to the core of identity, the loss of trust in expectations of oneself, of other persons, of one's society, and a reluctantly recognized questioning of meaning in the world—all these things combine to make experiences of shame almost impossible to communicate.

We may say, "I had an experience of such and such a sort," recounting its aspects which belong to some named class of experiences. But the minute, concrete detail—of inappropriate facial expression, bodily awkwardness, inept shading of voice, choice of word revealing Philistine taste, the particular manner of shortcoming, or of reaching out and meeting no response—the actual thorn in the wound, this, although seemingly the smallest part of the whole experience, is almost unbearable to admit to recollection or to express in words to another. The possibility of having to communicate to another person a past experience of shame may bring into throbbing awareness of detail what one has attempted to shroud in general phrases.[a]

A particular situation may give rise to guilt or to shame or to both. But guilt is more concerned with the codified act involved, shame with the uncodified detail and with the diffused feeling. Stealing a dime, killing a man, committing adultery, however vague or various the codes that cover them, are nevertheless specific acts of guilt which can be fitted into a more or less coherent scheme and which carry recognized consequences that can, to some extent at least, be anticipated. Nothing comparable covers lack of beauty or grace, errors of taste and congruence, weakness and certain kinds of failure, feelings of meanness or envy, rejection of the gift of oneself—situations that are experienced as exposure of deeply personal inadequacy.

Codes or conventions, says Conrad, provide ways of assorting, assimilating, and bearing experience.[a] Recognition of this use of ritual or convention is widespread. "Yet he took [his bitter personal defeat] with dignity; he even laid on it a certain ritual in order to keep it from being a low and shameful experience." [b]

For many people no experience can produce more disturbance than that that fits into no discernible pattern. The association of shame with confounding and confusion and the use of familiar detail to surmount experiences of shame emphasize this common human phenomenon. The contemporary existence of *anomie,* literally being without a norm, has engaged the attention of such sociologists as Emile Durkheim and Robert K. Merton because, according to Merton's hypothesis, contemporary society with its "disassociation between culturally prescribed aspirations and socially structured avenues for realizing these aspirations" brings about deviant, uncodified behavior. Imperfect co-ordination of goals and means in society leads to *anomie.*[c] Naming, structure, social norms, ritualized detail, and closure or correspondence between stated cultural goals and ways of realizing them give security and protection. Except for the person sufficiently deep-rooted in his own identity to be freely exploring, whatever cannot be codified, classified, labeled is potentially threatening, and can lead to a sense of being lost, unconnected. The wood in *Through the Looking-Glass* where no creature bears a name is a place of terror.

It has been frequently pointed out that it is harder to recount daydreams than those that occur in sleep. In daydreams we retain or can recapture consciousness and therefore feel more personally responsible for these fantasies than for dreams that occur in sleep. There is no widely recognized pattern or explanation of waking fantasies that lifts the weight of personal responsibility.[d] The difference of feeling about waking and sleeping dreams has perhaps been accentuated since Freud has provided names and a code into which dreams in sleep can be fitted.

Shame sets one apart. There is no clear code of shame. Voluntarily or involuntarily, one has opened oneself and the openness has been misunderstood or rejected; there has been weakness and failure in one's own eyes. Guilt, at least in our culture, can be a form of communication. There is communication of a sort not only between penitent and confessor, but between criminal and judge. Condemnation or punishment is itself a form of communication, relation to one's fellows. It fits in; it gives a code to cling to even if one has violated it. Hawthorne says of Hester Prynne, "The very law that condemned her . . . had held her up through the terrible ordeal of her ignominy." [a] Punishment merited by a guilty act or even undeserved punishment for an act one has not committed may be a refuge from shame.[b] In the midst of a situation in which one is overwhelmed by shame one may confess to a crime of which one is innocent, inviting punishment in order to re-establish, even through condemnation, communication with others.[c]

The very fact that shame is an isolating experience also means that if one can find ways of sharing and communicating it this communication can bring about particular closeness with other persons and with other groups. This can become the situation with minority groups or with minority positions in a particular historical situation. What is directed against a group as a label of shame can be converted into a mark of honor, and the group itself gains in strength.

There is no readily expressive language of shame, of identity, of mutuality, no accepted form by which these experiences can be communicated. Rebecca West believes that communication of such "living" experiences is impossible.

> There is no such thing as conversation. . . . There are intersecting monologues, that is all. We speak; we spread round us with sounds, with words, an emanation from ourselves. Sometimes they overlap the circles that others are spreading around themselves. . . . I am talking now of times when life is being lived . . . not when the intellect is holding the field. Then, of course, ideas can be formulated . . . like handing round a pearl on which you wish an opinion to a circle of experts. You cup the palm to hold it, you keep the hand very steady. No such caution is possible when one is really living. Then there is no conversation.[d]

Lack of a language may contribute to a sense of estrangement. Carson McCullers describes the effort to reach other people with words.

> F. Jasmine could not speak the unknown words, so after a minute she knocked her head a last time on the door and then began to walk around the kitchen table. . . . She began to talk in a high fast voice, but they were the wrong words, and not what she had meant to say.[a]

Contrasting the emotional concomitants of shame and guilt, Piers says that the unconscious, irrational threat implied in shame anxiety is abandonment, in contrast to the fear in guilt of mutilation.

> Behind the feeling of shame stands not the fear of hatred, but the fear of contempt which . . . spells fear of abandonment . . . the deeper rooted shame anxiety is based on the fear of the parent who walks away "in disgust," and . . . this anxiety in turn draws its terror from the earlier established and probably ubiquital separation anxiety.[b]

Important as is Piers' emphasis on the different kinds of anxieties that are the outcome of shame and guilt, it seems to me probable that the anguish of the experience of shame is not so much the fear that isolation or alienation will be the *penalty* for the shameful act as that the experience of shame is itself isolating, alienating, incommunicable.

A small child allowed to play with the loom of an older girl cut all the strings of the loom to remove her weaving and, when questioned, lied about having done this. There was certainly guilt over having destroyed the loom by cutting the strings and over having lied about it; but deeper than this, I believe, there was shame over the fact that she had cut the strings trustingly, in good faith, thinking that that was the way to remove the pattern, not knowing that it would damage the loom. The discovery left her alone and bewildered. The lie covered her inability to communicate the trust that had been shattered and the confused doubt that replaced it.

Being isolated, cut off, unable to find any way of being recognized by oneself and others as part of humanity is a peculiarly frightening experience. Donne's perception of this may be one reason that lines from Donne appear as titles or themes of so many novels in this present time of awareness of isolation.

As Sicknes is the greatest misery, so the greatest misery of sicknes is *solitude.* . . . *Solitude* is a torment which is not threatened in *hell* it selfe. Meere *vacuitie* the first *Agent,* God . . . will not admit; Nothing can be utterly *emptie;* but so neere a degree towards *Vacuitie* as *Solitude,* to bee but one, they [God and Nature] love not.[a]

For persons with certain forms of brain injury the desire for human identity is so great and the need to avoid isolation so strong that a person will go to almost any lengths to maintain the first and avoid the second.[b] Using Piers' contrast between consequences of guilt and shame, we recognize that one can exist and retain one's identity even if mutilated. If sufficiently isolated, estranged, one may question one's own existence.

When the threat of isolation is acute the need of establishing some sort of relationship is so great that there is an attempt to break through the barriers by any means however false or inadequate. In the extreme isolation of approaching schizophrenia a person desperately grasps any signals that it is thought "They" may understand:

One day we were jumping rope . . . when it came my turn and I saw my partner jump toward me. . . . I was seized with panic; I did not recognize her. . . . Standing at the other end of the rope, she had seemed smaller, but the nearer we approached each other . . . the more she swelled in size.

I cried out, "Stop, Alice, you look like a lion; you frighten me!" . . . I tried to dissemble [my fear] under the guise of fooling . . . actually, I didn't see a lion at all: it was only an attempt to describe the enlarging image of my friend and the fact that I didn't recognize her.[c]

Even in more usual predicaments a person sometimes adopts a means of communication that he thinks "They" may understand when he can find no way of expressing what is to him the reality. Collingwood describes the means he adopted in boyhood to pacify the adults when he was wrestling with "a formless and aimless intellectual disturbance" that he could not name.

> I know now that this is what always happens when I am in the early stages of work on a problem. Until the problem has gone a long way towards being solved, I do not know what it is . . . anyone who observed me must have thought, as my elders did think, that I had fallen into a habit of loafing. . . . My only defence against this opinion . . . was to cover these fits of abstraction with some bodily activity, trifling enough not to distract my attention from my inward wrestling. . . . So when the fit was upon me I would set myself to make something quite uninteresting, like a regiment of paper men. . . . It was painful to be laughed at for playing with paper men; but the alternative, to explain why I did it, was impossible.[a]

Awareness of loneliness, of isolation, is one of the most characteristic experiences of the contemporary world. Marx's chief condemnation of capitalism is that it alienates the individual.[b] The phenomenon of individual isolation is a cornerstone of existentialist philosophy, and the fact of alienation in the contemporary world is one thing that gives existentialism its contemporary appeal.[c] Freud regards separation and fear of separation as one of the main factors in anxiety.[d] The situation of isolation is a central theme in Fromm's *Escape from Freedom,*[e] in Sullivan's psychology of interpersonal relations, and in Durkheim's and Merton's analysis of *anomie.*

The search for ways to transcend loneliness pervades much contemporary writing, and the study of different kinds and degrees of isolation engages much attention in recent social science. It is possible that this indicates more belief in the possibilities of communication and personal relations, less acceptance of the finality of individual estrangement, than was characteristic of the generation of Chekhov or even of Proust.

Estrangement and betrayal and ways of meeting them constantly recur as themes in Graham Greene's novels. Portrayal of loneliness and of ways of overcoming it is central in the work of Carson McCullers and helps to explain her wide appeal. Of F. Jasmine she says, "She was not afraid of Germans or bombs or Japanese. She was afraid because in the war they would not include her, and because the world seemed somehow separate from herself." [a]

Elizabeth Bowen describes the search for a language in which the deepest, most individual experiences can be expressed:

> Innocence so constantly finds itself in a false position that inwardly innocent people learn to be disingenuous. Finding no language in which to speak in their own terms, they resign themselves to being translated imperfectly. They exist alone; when they try to enter into relations they compromise falsifyingly—through anxiety, through desire to impart and to feel warmth. . . . They are bound to blunder, then to be told they cheat. . . .[b]

Virginia Woolf herself felt, and also expressed through the characters with whom she identified, the conflict between wanting to come out of isolation and hesitancy to trust herself to communication. "Her strength and her limitations were that she didn't know really how it felt to be someone else. What she did know was how it felt to be alone, unique, isolated. . . ."[c]

> After all [Katharine] considered, why should she speak? Because it is right, her instinct told her; right to expose oneself without restraint to other human beings. She flinched from the thought. . . . Something she must keep of her own. But if she did keep something of her own? Immediately she figured an immured life . . . the same feeling living for ever, neither dwindling nor changing within the ring of a thick stone wall. The imagination of this loneliness frightened her.[d]

Protection against isolation and the difficulty of communicating such experiences as shame may take the form of impersonalization and dehumanization. If I cannot communicate with others, then I will at least not risk openness; I will deny the possibility of openness; I will protect myself against it.*

> K. had a large room in the Bank with a waiting-room attached to it and could watch the busy life of the city through his enormous plate-glass window.[e]

* See pp. 184-93 for further discussion of contemporary forms of protection against vulnerability through depersonalization.

Discussing Maupassant's protective plate glass of impersonality V. S. Pritchett says:

> It is impossible to know what hardens the heart, what checks the impulse to "look inside." . . . We can surmise that the broken home of the Maupassants had fixed the detachment, the watchfulness, the habit of *surveillance* in the child. . . . It is the outside that must be watched and . . . the very title of *Le Horla*—what is outside—shows that the horrors come from *an outside world that cannot be trusted* . . . this was Maupassant's terror: that the world would crash inwards upon a nature that . . . could not make itself hard, efficient, drastic, sealed off, and settled enough . . . he was at home only in the disconnected episode.[a] (Italics mine.)

> As one of his letters says: "Men, women or events—they mean nothing to me. I don't even care about myself." Life, he decided, was meaningless; it is a philosophy that leaves the door wide open for loneliness, melancholy—and personal push.[b]

The difficulty of communicating experiences of shame and the markedly different ways of responding to such experiences suggest that they can lead in two different directions: 1. They can lead to protection of the exposed self and of the exposed society at all costs—refusing to recognize the wound, covering the isolating effect of shame through depersonalization and adaptation to any approved codes. 2. If experiences of shame can be fully faced, if we allow ourselves to realize their import, they can inform the self, and become a revelation of oneself, of one's society, and of the human situation.

In attempts to understand diffused experiences of which shame is one example the development of a language that can express such experiences becomes of great importance. Certain current methods in the study of personality may hamper, not help, the creation of such a language. Other emerging methods may contribute more toward it. These different approaches to the study of personality will be the subject of the next two chapters.

THREE

Contemporary Study of Personality

If experiences of shame, with some such characteristics as I have suggested, may be deeply revealing of the self and of the social situation, it becomes important to ask why shame has been neglected in study. Consideration of certain habits of thought, "codifications of reality," in Dorothy Lee's words, that underlie much contemporary psychology and social science suggest reasons for the lack of attention given to shame—as well as to other experiences that are profound and difficult to communicate.

Some of these ways of thinking, these conscious or unconscious assumptions, are so embedded in our language and in our concepts that we tend to regard them, not as interpretations of reality, but as attributes of reality itself. They permeate theories of personality as different as those of Freud and Pavlov. In our careful delineation of the differences between psychoanalysis and academic psychology and among various schools of each, we frequently overlook the extent to which their different theories of personality development share assumptions, analogies, or idioms that set an unrecognized framework within which their observations and theories are shaped.

Certain of these forms of thought seem to us so inescapable that it scarcely occurs to us that there could be any radically different ways of phrasing reality. A theory developed to refute a particular theory may be simply an alternate position based on the same premises, an acceptance of the terms in which the problem is to be studied. In some theories these terms are explicitly stated in a formal scheme which aims at nothing less than logical completeness, a comprehensive set of categories within which all aspects of personality and culture are to be accommodated. In others, the assumptions are unstated but are implicit in the metaphors and concepts used in describing the human enterprise.

The account of certain prevailing ways of thought and study presented in this chapter should not be read as implying that these approaches to reality are bad, and that the newer ones described in the next chapter are good. Each view mentioned here has contributed greatly to our understanding and will continue to do so. The question is by no means one of replacing them, but of supplementing them in order to gain more insight into forms of behavior that they tend to miss.

In pointing out certain of the basic presuppositions or axioms that affect schools of contemporary thought widely different from one another, I am clearly not attempting to give anything like an adequate account of any particular presupposition, still less of any particular school. Rather, I am simply suggesting certain modes of thought that tend to be taken for granted even when the attempt is made to develop a new conceptual scheme, new experimental methods, or a new vocabulary.

Thinking from Parts to Wholes

In our study of personality and society we characteristically work from parts to wholes, attempting to discover discrete items of behavior, then adding them together and trying to find relations among them. It is taken for granted that the units accessible to understanding are series of elements, items, or particulars that can be classified into groups. Part and whole are, of course, both relative concepts; everything is a part relative to something more comprehensive and a whole relative to something less so. But until recently a strong tendency in Western thought has been to assume that truth is to be found by breaking down observed phenomena into smaller and smaller parts and measuring these parts more and more accurately. This has been truer of psychology than of sociology and perhaps anthropology, since psychology sought more rigorously to model itself on the methods of the natural science of the nineteenth century, while such sociologists as Herbert Spencer and Auguste Comte were more influenced by what they thought were the sweeping conclusions of the natural sciences.

Some psychologists believe that the sequence of thinking from supposedly discrete entities to larger wholes is no longer dominant, that the differences between atomistic and holistic psychology have been largely reconciled or resolved in favor of holistic or *Gestalt* concepts.[a] In the writings of many contemporary sociologists there is an effort to distinguish and combine concepts of different degrees of inclusiveness such as the individual, his immediate social group, and the wider society. And certainly the vocabulary of psychology has in the last fifteen or twenty years included more terms referring to larger units of study.* But the writings of both academic and psychoanalytic psychologists suggests that the actual shift in ways of thinking may not have been as great as the new terms would seem to indicate. We may talk of holism, of field theory, of the necessity of seeing details in a *Gestalt* and still continue to think in atomistic ways.

The emphasis on discrete entities as either the given or as that which it is most important to discover has a long history in Western thought. If an observation of Aristotle's did not fit into a named class of phenomena, he created a new classification. Aristotelian logic is embedded in our concepts and in our language. "European languages in general begin with a subject-noun whose action is expressed in an active verb. Some apparently permanent element is separated from the general process, treated as an entity, and endowed with active responsibility for a given occurrence. This procedure is so paradoxical that only long acquaintance with it conceals its absurdity." [b]

Hume revived an earlier tradition besides providing a prototype for contemporary positivism in his insistence that we can

* See discussion of the different uses of molar and molecular and of holistic concepts, pp. 126-32.

know only the separate elements of experience. On this ground he based his denial of the existence of a self.

> There are some philosophers who imagine we are every moment intimately conscious of what we call our *self*. . . .
> For my part, when I enter most intimately into what I call *myself*, I always stumble on some particular perception or other, of heat or cold, light or shade, love or hatred, pain or pleasure. I never can catch *myself* at any time without a perception, and never can observe anything but the perception. When my perceptions are removed for any time, as by sound sleep, so long am I insensible of *myself*. . . . They [mankind] are nothing but a bundle or collection of different perceptions.[a]

Hume could not discover the self because he was looking for another element or separate perception like heat or cold; his method of observation and analysis precluded the possibility of reaching a more comprehensive concept.[b] Thus to Hume the concepts of shame and the sense of identity as pervasive experiences would have been without basis in reality and without valid meaning.

The logic of John Stuart Mill, in the wake of Hume, tended to treat all psychological problems as soluble by an atomistic, associationist psychology. F. H. Bradley revolted against this form of atomism, the analysis of a judgment into detachable terms that are prior to propositions. He maintained that a thought is a functional unity, possessing distinguishable features but not composed of detachable pieces, and that a proposition cannot be said to be true or false because of self-consistency, but must have objective reference.[c]

A distinction must be made here between atomism and specification. Atomism refers to the assumption that the universe is composed of simple, indivisible, and minute units externally related to each other. Specification refers to the necessity of saying as clearly as we can what it is that we are investigating. The necessity to specify shades into a theory of atomism if it includes the implicit assumption that the smaller and more isolable the units into which phenomena can be broken down the clearer and more precise specifications can be, and the closer we can come to reality. It is this implicit assumption that has characterized much of the development of Western science and that is currently open to question.

The terms determinate and indeterminate variables have come to be used in psychological and social-scientific writing to signify those units that are regarded for purposes of a particular study as fixed and under control and those that are regarded as not under control and therefore subject to testing and experiment. Whatever terms we use we must make clear what we are starting with, what we are trying to find out, what we regard as under control, and what is not under control but "free" to respond for purposes of a particular study. The necessity of such distinctions is not in question. What is in question is what kinds of phenomena may be habitually excluded from study by those items that are customarily singled out for control and for study; what is excluded by starting, to the extent that we usually do, with the small and discrete and supposedly fixed items, and demanding clarity and precision in such items. Much depends upon what questions we ask, what we consider as givens in an inquiry, and what is to be discovered. We cannot know whether a proposition is true or false without knowing, not only its relation to the external world, but what question it is trying to answer.

The assumption that understanding proceeds by means of first seeking the discrete, supposedly unchanging elements into which a phenomenon under study can be analyzed and only later turning attention to the changes going on in the elements and to the relations among them is still very much with us. Sumner's statement that "from the first acts by which men try to satisfy needs each act stands by itself and looks no further than the immediate satisfaction" [a] is out of date, if at all, in its manner of expression rather than in its underlying thought.

The methods of John Whiting are a particularly marked, but not an uncharacteristic, example of the use of this assumption. A scientific hypothesis is to him a tentative statement of the relation between two separate units or events; in validating a hypothesis it is necessary to isolate antecedent and consequent, and in the study of personality and culture understanding is reached by correlation of such isolates. Units of individual behavior are sought; and having started out with such separate units as given he reaches, by a chain of circular reasoning, the conclusion that "the practices of a society for one system of behavior are almost entirely independent of its practices with respect to other systems of behavior"; "aspects of child training practices . . . grow . . . out of antecedents specific to each system of behavior." [a] Integration of personality and culture in theory takes place after an initial assumption of separation.

For Parsons and Shils in their study that looks toward a general theory of human behavior[b] the place to start is with the isolation of certain specified units of behavior, regarded as if they were completely independent of each other and unchanging.[c] This assumption of separation and changelessness is necessary in order to meet their requirements of a good theory. Only after the study of the state of a system at a given moment has been completed should the study of the network of relations and of change in time be undertaken. The units of study are unaltered when viewed as isolated and unchanging and when viewed as related and in process of change. "There is . . . no difference between the variables involved in description of the state of a system and analysis of its processes. The difference lies in how the same variables are used." [d]

It is recognized that this separation and disregarding of change is an abstraction from the actual behavior of actual human beings, but it is looked upon as an abstraction necessary for scientific study. It is an inconvenience for science that the way human beings do behave interferes with this treatment of units of behavior as separate and static. In outlining ways to study the effect of maternal punishment on the aggression of the child and the effect of aggression on the punishment, Robert R. Sears says:

> Logically, and practically, a good theory requires that antecedents and consequents be entirely independent of one another. It would be most satisfactory if the child did not influence the mother's behavior, and if we could then say something about the effect of punishment on later behavior.[e]

The fact that the behavior of mother and child cannot empirically be so isolated from each other creates, as Sears is careful to state, a difficult research problem.

Parsons in his *Social System* and Parsons and Shils in their later study discuss the concepts of equilibrium, of process, and of dynamics—all of which present difficulties to any investigator. Parsons' definition of equilibrium as a "boundary-maintaining" system[a] seems to me useful in emphasizing the necessity of at least a minimum of adaptation, self-preservation, and continuity if a phenomenon is to remain recognizably itself. Process seems to be used in the more usual sense of any changes occurring in a phenomenon or in related phenomena over a period of time, and in a somewhat more specialized sense as "any way or mode in which a given state of a system or of a part of a system changes into another state." [b] There is recognition that the word dynamic sometimes carries unstated assumptions that dynamic refers particularly to motives or to development or sometimes to unconscious processes.[c] But Parsons refers to most social systems as "dynamically changing," [d] without making entirely clear what his use of dynamic adds to the concept of process or change.

It is easier to observe many objects or events as if they were unchanging than to observe the processes in which they are always involved. But it does not follow from this relative ease of observation that equilibrium is a more normal or basic or important aspect of a phenomenon or system of phenomena than is change.* Parsons and Shils recognize that all individual and group behavior is constantly changing and that the dynamics (the energy or causal factors) of change is sooner or later necessary for any study of behavior; and Parsons is at pains to defend his structural-functional theory of society from charges of being static.[e] But it is not without significance that factors making for maintaining equilibrium come first in this analysis and factors making for change second and that there is assumed to be "no difference between the variables involved in description of the state of a system and analysis of its processes." [f]

One question raised by this way of thinking is whether logical

* See Kurt Goldstein on this point and further discussion of process, pp. 133-40.

completeness is a desirable aim at this stage of our empirical knowledge. Study of change may interfere with logical completeness. Process is less readily observed in some phenomena, objects, or events than in others. But change in time can never be ignored or forgotten or added on as a relatively extraneous factor; it is always present. What are called structures in biology, for example, may be regarded as slow processes of long duration, what are called functions as more rapid processes of short duration.[a]

If the separate atoms or items linked together furnish manifestly inadequate explanations of human behavior, the tendency is not to re-examine the method but to create new links in the chain. Thus to independent variables and dependent variables are added hypothetical intervening variables; ". . . the need system is to be thought of as a set of interconnecting compartments, each compartment corresponding to a differentiated need." [b] It is possible as an outcome of present habits of thought to speak of the need of a "*rapprochement*" between the "*field* of personality, *on the one hand,*" and the "*field* of perception, *on the other.*" [c] (Italics mine.)

All this suggests that our training inclines us to comprehend a totality of relations or a continuing process of change only after it has first been broken up into items or smaller categories. We give names to forms, structures, and functions rather than to more diffused, changing experiences.

Dorothy Lee calls this preoccupation with proceeding from parts to wholes, from separate items to integration, from isolated events to cause-and-effect sequences and changes, a lineal codification of reality that differs from the nonlineal codifications of reality employed by certain other cultures.* She describes our way of constantly acting in terms of an implied line (in *drawing* a conclusion, *tracing* a relationship, *leading to* conclusions or a goal, taking *a course* of action, following the direction of an argument).[d] She contrasts this parts-to-whole, lineal characteristic of our thinking with the thought patterns of other

* Cf. discussion of Sapir's, Whorf's, and Hoijer's theories of the way the various patterns of language lead to the stressing of certain aspects of reality and ignoring of others differently in different societies, pp. 171-81.

peoples who select different aspects of reality for emphasis: the Ontang Javanese have words for emotional experiences but not for observed forms or functions; the Trobriands emphasize a patterned whole, not causal relationships or steps toward a climax,[a] the Wintu regard the given as an unpartitioned mass rather than as a series of particulars, and the individual as a differentiated part of society rather than society as a plurality of individuals.[b] A lineal codification of reality with stress on discrete items undoubtedly has been a major factor in the development of Western science. But it may be that making other kinds of experience accessible to understanding, and further development of science itself, requires an expansion of this way of thought.

Post-quantum developments in physics and recent work in biology suggest the inadequacy of the simpler lineal cause-and-effect concepts of the nineteenth century. Much psychological—perhaps less sociological—thought, however, still follows the concepts of an earlier physics and biology. We tend to take for granted separate events and objects and then attempt to trace connections and relations among them.

This parts-to-whole, lineal approach applied to the study of personality means that parts of the personality are regarded as separate units and then, the separation having been initially assumed, the problems of relation and integration are posed. The earlier segmenting of the personality into sensation, perception, and will, or listed traits and instincts has been replaced in Freudian and neo-Freudian thinking by segmenting into id, ego, and superego; unconscious, preconscious, and conscious. But the newer divisions, also, are often used as if they were discrete and isolable.

Anna Freud and other contemporary Freudians have come to take for granted the existence of id, ego, and superego as separate entities, and then go through elaborate explanations as to how these separate existences are related to each other. So distinct are they that Anna Freud can say, "the analyst . . . when he sets about the work of enlightenment . . . takes his stand at a point equidistant from the id, the ego, and the super-ego." [c] The "ego" ceases to be a metaphor or a part of a hypothesis and becomes an entity "independent of the emotions," a distinct and separate part of the personality.[a]

Ways of studying personality with less emphasis on the autonomy of separate parts, more on the functioning whole, will be discussed in the next chapter. It must be borne in mind, however, that the study of the whole does not make the study of subsystems unnecessary. Finer specification continues to be important. The point is that relations should be as much taken for granted and regarded as basic in the personality as separate items.

A similar assumed apartness and then laborious putting together occurs in our way of studying the individual *and* society. Here we are still influenced by post-Renaissance thinking, which takes as given separate individual human atoms and then poses as a problem how they can be related in society; by the Hobbesian view, which sees society as an aggregate of self-contained individuals, assimilated through some external instrument such as the common law. The separateness is assumed; the relationship is to be constructed. We discuss the necessity of combining individual behavior and social behavior into a single theoretical system[b] and the effect of culture on personality.[c] This separation is not accepted without question. The phrasing "personality *in* culture" is beginning to replace "personality *and* culture." [d] But, for people trained as many of us are, it is still difficult to think in terms other than those of separate individual atoms linked together in society.

A special instance of atomistic, lineal thinking is the stress on polarities, opposite ends of a scale, mutually exclusive opposites in Plato's sense, forms of thought used almost axiomatically in much psychological writing. Ernest Jones notes Freud's constant proclivity toward dualistic ideas; any kind of pluralism was alien to him. Throughout his professional life, Freud tended to think in terms of polarities: subject-object, the polarity of reality; pleasure-unpleasure, an economic polarity; active-passive, a biological polarity.[e]

Literary and artistic pursuits, says Melvin H. Marx, are at the "opposite end of the scale" from scientific method.[f] Books on personality abound in parallel columns of supposedly antithetical descriptive terms, and the word versus is frequently used to separate paired terms that are regarded as opposed rather than complementary to each other. We find such supposed antitheses in the use of active vs. passive, gratifying vs. noxious, need-gratifying vs. need-blocked, subject vs. object, pleasure vs. pain, dominance vs. submission, love vs. hate, friend vs. enemy, masculine vs. feminine.[a]

Psychological and Moral Scarcity

Methods of studying personality still rest on assumptions and make use of models derived from nineteenth-century Newtonian science and from classical economics. This was notably true of Freud, but it is also true of some psychologists who take sharp issue with fundamentals of Freudian theory. Freud's unresting search and his own thought constantly went beyond his models, but this has been less true of some who have been influenced by him.*

Freud, as Jones has made clear, modeled his theory of personality on the science of his youth. This meant the physiology of Bruecke and Helmholtz, both strongly influenced by nineteenth-century physics. Freud's physiology and his psychology in turn were thus conceived in terms of a physics of systems of atoms moved by forces, of conservation of energy, of relatively simple, lineal causation and determinism, of the belief that all phenomena are susceptible to specific quantitative treatment.[b]

In seeking functional and dynamic explanations, Freud went far beyond the more mechanical aspects of the Helmholtz school, but he never entirely dispensed with the earlier physiological principles. He was influenced by Darwin, but leaned more than Darwin did toward the Lamarckian theory of the inheritance of acquired characteristics.[c] He believed, not only that there is no evidence of psychical processes occurring apart from physiological ones, but that physical processes must precede psychical ones. He regarded men as phenomena of the physical world, and his desire was to express psychical processes

* See p. 88 n.

in terms of physiological processes, and physiological processes in terms of those of physics and chemistry,[a] ". . . to create a mind-robot, a thinking machine." [b] Freud's genius made his great discoveries relatively independent of his physical model. But the thinking of and the possibility of new discovery by many of his followers has shown more tendency to be cramped by the model. In biological science certain schemes and models based on nineteenth-century mechanistic theories of science still exert perhaps undue influence,[c] and this tends to be even truer in psychology.

The Newtonian principles that gave rise to nineteenth-century natural science also helped to shape nineteenth-century classical economics. Although Freud was not consciously influenced by economic theory as he was by physical science, his choice of language, of metaphor and analogy, naturally grew out of the prevailing thought of his time.

The basic analogy of Freud's theory of personality is a quantitative analogy of economic distribution. This economic analogy certainly grew more refined and specialized in Freud's later development of his theory, and was more influenced by the dynamic and topological aspects of the theory.[d] But the central economic analogy persists, and, as in its classical model, the economics is an economics of scarcity. Freud constantly makes use of such terms as the economy of the personality and the quantity of energy that can be distributed. Basic to his thinking is a libido-fund theory analogous to the wage-fund theory. There is a limited amount of money, or of psychic energy, to be distributed; it can be redistributed and obstacles to its maximum or optimum distribution can be removed, but it cannot be enhanced or enriched.

This libido-fund theory is one of the concepts that was not altered in essentials with the development of other aspects of Freud's thought:

> . . . We thus formulate . . . the concept of a *libido-quantum*.[e]

> We perceive . . . a certain reciprocity between ego-libido and object-libido. The more that is absorbed by the one, the more impoverished does the other become. The highest form of . . . object-

libido is . . . being in love, when the subject seems to yield up his whole personality in favor of object cathexis. . . .[a]

At the same time the ego has put forth its libidinal object-cathexes. It becomes *impoverished* in consequence both of these cathexes and of the formation of the ego-ideal, and it *enriches* itself again both by gratification of its object-love and by fulfilling its ideal.[b] (Italics mine.)

. . . as our knowledge increases we are ever being impelled to bring the *economic* point of view into the foreground.[c]

The term *"traumatic"* has actually no other meaning, but this *economic* one . . . lasting disturbances must result in the distribution of the available energy in the mind.[d]

In his last work, Freud says:

. . . the normal and abnormal phenomena that we observe . . . require to be described from the point of view of dynamics and of economics (*i.e.,* in this connection, from the point of view of the quantitative distribution of the libido.)[e]

Many contemporary Freudians object to the literal use of Freudian analogies, but they themselves for the most part continue to use the basic economic analogy and the concept of a limited fund of psychic energy. Thus Therese Benedek says:

Receiving, retaining, eliminating—taking and giving—regulate the physiologic and psychic economy all through life.[f]

Fortunate is the man whose primary emotional gratifications keep balance with the spending of psychic and physical energies in work. Even the gratifications of secondary narcissism [in work] may become a steady drain upon the psychic resources, leaving but little libido for primary emotional gratification.[g]

The same economics of scarcity as applied to psychic energy appears in David Rapaport's theories of the development of the ego and of thought. These are based on Freud's economics of cathectic energy.* Rapaport, following Freud, holds that only

* Cathexis is literally a charge or investment of energy; more specifically, in Parsons and Shils' definition, attachment to objects that give pleasure, avoidance or rejection of those that give pain. "Freud thought of the process whereby an external stimulus (object) comes to elicit an instinctual response as analogous

a limited amount of energy is available to the ego. It follows that when a certain amount of energy is employed to make certain ideas conscious it must of necessity be withdrawn from other ideas.[a]

Among non-Freudians the influence of nineteenth-century science and economics sometimes seems to persist in a tendency to reject as subjects for investigation any phenomena that do not lend themselves to observation, to relatively simple theories of causation, and to quantitative treatment. Glenn Negley is perhaps too sweeping in his assertion that much contemporary theory in social science and psychology seems to assume that "quantification is the only acceptable method of observation and classification of data, that more precise quantification of data is *ipso facto* more complete and precise description of data, and finally, that no data which are not quantifiable can be the proper subject of observation and description." [b] But certainly many statements on experiment and quantification by contemporary psychologists and social scientists seem to lend themselves to this interpretation.*

The use of an economic idiom as a basic analogy applies not only to ways of studying personality, but, very widely, to theories of personality and of society. There is a tendency to see all human behavior as a matter of quantitative exchange of scarce commodities. What Erich Fromm has called this market-place

---

to the manner in which a neutral physical object acquires an electrical charge and behaves as if it were an electrical force. This process is called cathecting. An object or even a complex reaction pattern may be cathected—*i.e.*, acquire 'charge' from the original instinctual drive." (Ruth Monroe, *Schools of Psychoanalytic Thought*, Dryden Press, 1955, p. 97n.)

* B. F. Skinner, for example, contends that a science of human behavior has little to gain from using concepts of psychic events that have different dimensions from the dimensions of physical science. He says, "The objection to inner states is not that they do not exist but that they are not relevant to a functional analysis." Behavior cannot be assumed to have any properties that call for unique methods of study. Skinner rules out such words as meaning, intent, understanding. (Samuel M. Strong, review of B. F. Skinner, *Science and Human Behavior*, New York, Macmillan, 1953, *American Journal of Sociology*, Vol. LX, No. 3, Nov. 1954, p. 323.)

Cf. pp. 143-6 for criticism by Gordon Allport, Henry A. Murray, and others of some of these assumptions.

psychology has been active in Western thought since the Commercial Revolution, and especially since the Industrial Revolution. George Eliot recognized it in early nineteenth-century England:

> Poor Mr. Casaubon had imagined that his long studious bachelorhood had stored up for him a compound interest of enjoyment, and that large drafts on his affections would not fail to be honored . . . now he was in danger of being saddened by the very conviction that his circumstances were unusually happy: there was nothing external by which he could account for a certain blankness which came over him just when his expectant gladness should have been most lively.[a]

A comment on this characteristically Western view of the economy of personality appears in Forster's *A Passage to India.*

> [Fielding says] "Your emotions never seem in proportion to their objects, Aziz."
>
> "Is emotion a sack of potatoes, so much to the pound to be measured out? Am I a machine? I shall be told I shall use up my emotions by using them next."
>
> "I should have thought you would. It sounds common sense. You can't eat your cake and have it, even in the world of the spirit."
>
> "If you are right, there is no point in any friendship; it all comes down to give and take, or give and return, which is disgusting, and we had all better leap over this parapet and kill ourselves." [b]

Compensatory Theory of Personality Development

Related to the scarcity theory of psychic energy is the view that personality develops through a series of compensatory devices, which must overcome primary antisocial and undesirable tendencies. (Primary, in the vocabulary of psychology and of psychoanalysis, has several different meanings not always clearly distinguished: earlier in time, greater in strength and influence, of more lasting importance.) This compensatory theory of personality development extends from Freud and contemporary

Freudians to contemporary experimental learning-school theorists, and is far-reaching in its implications.*

According to it, a child is born with certain biological-psychological urges or drives into an environment (in any conceivable period of history or in any conceivable organization of society) that thwarts those drives. The developing personality is continuously *acted upon* by pressures from within and from without, which create tensions or conflicts from which the individual struggles to free himself. Conflict is an inescapable evil, associated with disorder, misery, and fear, to be reduced as much as possible.[a] To be "conflict-free" is desirable, although "a measure of frustration and conflict" is necessary for the development of such "personality *devices*" as the "higher thought processes, ideals, and conscience."[b] (Italics mine.) The individual remains largely passive except under pressure. The clue to personality development is found in the attempt of the individual to get freedom from specific pressures, release of specific tensions.

Some clarification of terms is necessary at this point. The words needs, drives, and goals are used by psychologists and psychoanalysts with a variety of different meanings and implications. All schools of psychoanalysis would say that individuals are "goal-directed." But goals as used in a compensatory theory of personality are limited, segmented, and narrowly related to particular needs; goal-directed means the attempt to satisfy these special needs, instead of having reference to any wider,

* The attempt to understand Freud, as well as Hartmann and other contemporary Freudians, presents the endlessly fascinatmg and difficult problem of trying to distinguish meaning from words, of trying to discern the central thrust of the thought of a creative person through the images and metaphors of his time in which he has almost inevitably expressed it. The same problem appears in a very different form in, for example, the attempt to enter into the meaning of George Herbert and the other metaphysical poets of the seventeenth century. They used the symbolism of the liturgy and the religious art of their time; but in using it they both enlarged the meaning of the symbols they used and used the symbols to enlarge their vision of the meaning of life. In reading Freud it is not easy to know when the metaphors and analogies that were those of his time constricted his thought. But there is no doubt that the power of his insights continues to unfold, and that it enlarges the meanings of the forms in which it was originally invested at the same time that it continues to seek more adequate means of expression.

long-term purposes of human beings. The only wider purpose is to restore an equilibrium. Restoration of equilibrium comprises the purposes of men and the possibilities of human development.*

Ruth Munroe's account of Freudian theory makes the useful point that the distinction between needs and drives is primarily a matter of emphasis in describing the same process, needs emphasizing the inner state and drives the direction of attention outward.[a] She also rightly stresses the range and variety of Freud's explanations and theories of causation. But, with all her stress on the multidimensional aspects of Freud's theory, she still uses goal as a limited specific object which is sought in order to reduce tension.[b]

Confining goals to specific objects, in the view of some psychologists, restricts unduly both the conception of human potentialities and of the nature of the external world. Andras Angyal, for example, believes that the concept of goal should be extended to include the active relation between subject and object, and between the satisfaction of a specific need and the deeper, more pervasive tendency of which this need is a manifestation.[c] It is questionable whether the limited use of goal as tension-releasing object can describe those activities that are most characteristically human. The human interests in exploring the world, in creative thought, in reaching out toward other persons cannot take place under too strong need-pressure with too narrow a goal.[d] Understanding of such an experience as shame requires a wider conception of goals and of human capacities.

It has been necessary to anticipate later discussion of other views in order to make clear the specific meaning of goal-directed in a compensatory theory of personality.†

Freud's thought is rooted in and shaped by a compensatory view of personality. It appears in his theories of personality de-

* The concept of equilibrium can be used to refer to a creation of an equilibrium of a different sort or on another level, but in Freud's thought the emphasis on restoration of a previous equilibrium is prominent.

† See pp. 147-52, 256 for elaboration of Schachtel's and other wider views of goal and purpose. Robert K. Merton believes that contemporary sociology does not follow Freud's compensatory or reductionist theories.

velopment, of the relations of human beings with each other, of the possibilities for the individual in society, of thought and the relation of human beings to the "reality" of the nonpersonal world.

On personality development:

Cruelty is intimately related to the childish character, since the *inhibition* which restrains the mastery impulse before it causes pain to others—*that is, the capacity for sympathy*—develops comparatively late.[a] (Italics mine.)

. . . all the feelings of sympathy, friendship, *trust* and so forth which we expend in life are genetically connected with sexuality and have developed out of purely sexual desires by *an enfeebling* of their sexual aim.[b] (Italics mine.)

. . . these praiseworthy and valuable qualities [generosity and kindheartedness] are based on *compensation* and *overcompensation* [for miserliness and unfriendliness].[c] (Italics mine.)

[The] chief function [of the superego] remains the *limitation* of satisfactions.[d]

[The] diversion [outward of the destructive instinct] . . . seems essential for the preservation of the individual. . . .[e]

. . . nature has given children to women as a substitute for the penis that has been denied them.[f]

On relations with other persons:

It is only when someone is completely in love that the main quantity of libido is transferred on to the object and the object *to some extent takes the place of* the ego.[g] (Italics mine.)

Parental love . . . is *nothing but* parental narcissism born again. . . .[h] (Italics mine.)

The time comes when every one of us has to abandon the illusory anticipation with which in our youth we regarded our fellow-men, and when we realize how much hardship and suffering we have been caused in life through their ill-will.[i]

According to Schopenhauer's famous simile of the freezing porcupine no one can tolerate too intimate an approach to his neighbor.

The evidence of psycho-analysis shows that almost every intimate relation between two people which lasts for some time—marriage, friendship, the relations between parents and children—leaves a sediment of feelings of aversion and hostility, which have first to be eliminated by repression.[a]

Social feeling is based upon the reversal of what was first a hostile feeling into a positively-toned tie of the nature of an identification.[b]

Freud sets the limits of the kinds of relationships that are possible between human beings:*

In the individual's mental life someone else is invariably involved, as a model, as an object, as a helper, as an opponent.[c]

On the individual in society:

Our civilization is, generally speaking, founded on the suppression of instincts. Each individual has contributed some renunciation—of his sense of dominating power, of the aggressive and vindictive tendencies of his personality.[d]

. . . the sense of guilt is the most important [factor] in the evolution of culture. . . . the price of progress . . . is . . . forfeiting happiness through heightening of the sense of guilt.[e]

. . . 'cultural privation' dominates the whole field of social relations between human beings; we know already that it is the cause of the antagonism against which all civilization has to fight.[f]

. . . this unconscious, in which all that is evil in the human mind is contained as a predisposition . . . 'dread of society' (*soziale Angst*) is the essence of what is called conscience.[g]

On Thought and the Nonpersonal World:

. . . the desire for knowledge . . . often gives one the impression that it can actually take the place of sadism in the mechanism of the obsessional neurosis. After all, it is at bottom an *off-shoot*, sublimated and raised to the intellectual sphere, *of the possessive* instinct. . . .[h] (Italics mine.)

* Freud himself found an intimate friend and a hated enemy always indispensable to his emotional life; he said that he always created them anew if they temporarily did not exist; sometimes they coincided in the same person. More than once he turned a close friend into an enemy. (Ernest Jones, *Sigmund Freud*, Hogarth Press, Vol. I, pp. 9, 177-8.)

> . . . an essential pre-condition for the institution of the function for testing reality is that objects *shall have been lost* [absent or delayed in appearance] which have formerly afforded real satisfaction. . . .[a] (Italics mine.)

> That which [man] projects ahead of him as his ideal is merely his substitution for the lost narcissism of his childhood. . . .[b]

These quotations from Freud are not isolated examples taken out of context. They represent a main stream of his thought.

Contemporary Freudians have extended in many directions, notably in the development of ego psychology, the modifications and elaborations of this theory made by Freud himself. But in general they have not altered the compensatory assumptions of the theory.

Thus, satisfaction in work is regarded as "secondary narcissism," the delights of motherhood as originating in "primarily introverted narcissistic tendencies," fatherhood as an urge "to conquer . . . dependent needs through heterosexual love," fantasy as "an intra-psychic safety valve which yields relief from tension and at the same time provides intermediary steps in development." [c] "Feelings of guilt . . . are a fundamental incentive towards creativeness and work . . . any source of joy, beauty and enrichment . . . is, in the unconscious mind, felt to be the mother's loving and giving breast and the father's creative penis. . . ." [d]

Heinz Hartmann has gone further perhaps than any other strict Freudian in recognizing independent and other than compensatory factors in the development of the ego and of thought. But, although he declares his intention to demonstrate the relative independence of ego development, and to show that "Learning to think and learning in general are independent biological functions which exist beside, and in part independently of, drives and defenses," an explanation of personality development as compensation still occupies a definite place in his thought.[e] He believes, for example, that the development from a sense of the objective world that exists only as long as it satisfies needs to a sense of the reality of objects existing independently of human needs comes about in part as the result of "neutralization of aggression." [f]

In paying tribute to Paul Schilder, Rapaport recognizes and approves Schilder's emphasis on the inviting nature of the real world and the indigenous curiosity and exploring quality of the human mind.[a] He quotes with approval Schilder's insistence that "human thinking is directed toward an existing world of objects . . . without assuming the existence [of which] no theory of thinking can be built," and that "socialization . . . is not an acquisition of thinking or human psychological life, but a basic implication of it." [b]

But in his comprehensive study *The Organization and Pathology of Thought,* Rapaport appears to lose interest in Schilder's insistence on man's naturally exploring attitude toward the world and to return to an almost exclusive emphasis on the Freudian "detour theory" of thinking. Thought in this view is a substitute for a desired object not immediately present. The "primary model" of thought is mounting drive-tension—absence of drive-object—hallucinatory image of it. "Secondary-process thought . . . does not accept or reject according to immediate pleasure or pain, but seeks the pleasurable object—that is, the tension relieving, the gratifying—by detours. . . . Thought . . . show[s] the safest way to tension-release." [c]

Even with the most brilliant contemporary exponents and amplifiers of the Freudian theory, such as Hartmann and Rapaport, the acceptance of a basically compensatory theory of personality development gives rise to an elaborate series of double negatives to account for positive, purposive aspects of human behavior. Thus Rapaport, following Ernst Kris, gives this description of the process of creative thought:

> When an unconscious idea rises to consciousness, the ego suspends its censoring function momentarily, only to resume it again. . . . In terms of energy-dynamics: the *countercathectic* energy-distributions become momentarily *ineffective,* and part of their energy is probably used to hypercathect *the arising repressed idea.*[d] (Italics mine.)

In Hartmann's discussions of the relatively autonomous ego and Rapaport's discussion of the development of thought and judgments of the real world, such terms as the following abound: substitute gratifications, defense mechanisms, countercathexis, secondary processes, quasi needs, coping with reality, displacement, substitution, ideas as safety valves of drive tension, ego-regression in love and creative thought.[a]

So blinding can a compensatory theory of personality be that it has recently come as a surprise to some psychologists and psychoanalysts to discover that children like to move! This fact once discovered, however, is considered of sufficient importance to merit a psychological christening. It now has a name—"primary motility." *

Explanations of humor and laughter offer peculiarly sensitive indexes to the dynamics and central animus of theories of personality. The Freudian and Neo-Freudian accounts of humor epitomize the compensatory theory of personality. Identical situations of suddenly perceived discrepancy or incongruity may, as noted above, be experienced as shameful or as ludicrous. What determines the difference?

The Freudian explanation (which can be traced to Plato and Aristotle) is easy. The difference lies in whether it is oneself or another who is unexpectedly exposed. In shame a person is seen around; in laughter he sees around others.[b]

According to this view, laughter occurs when there is a redistribution of the limited fund of psychic energy so that weakness, inferiority, or aggression may be *compensated for* by humor. Laughter or humor occur as realization of one's own power in relation to, or over, other people. In this sense they are exploitative of other people. Freud agrees with Hobbes that "*Sudden Glory,* is the passion which maketh those *grimaces* called LAUGHTER; and is caused either by some sudden act of their own, that pleaseth them; or by the apprehension of some deformed thing in another, by comparison whereof they suddenly applaud themselves." [c]

* Bela Mittelmann, who has given much attention to "motility," notes that in earlier psychoanalytic formulations the movement of children has been dealt with as (a) a component of the sexual instinct (at times referred to as muscle eroticism); (b) an executive function, largely under conscious control; (c) a means, or possibly a source, of aggression (sadism); (d) an avenue of tension discharge; (e) in play a way of overcoming anxiety. ("Motility in Infants, Children, and Adults," *Psychoanalytic Study of the Child,* Vol. IX, 1954, p. 142.) At least four of these formulations appear to be versions of a compensatory theory of personality.

The late Ernst Kris, the leading recent exponent of the Freudian theory of humor, stresses the kinship between Freud and Hobbes.[a] Kris' explanations of humor rest upon concepts of both scarcity of psychic energy and compensation for defects:

Laughter breaks out . . . when a sum of psychic energy which has been employed for the cathexis of certain psychic trends suddenly becomes unusable.[b]

. . . the saving in mental energy which accompanies caricature . . . is evidently to be regarded as a saving in expenditure on suppression, or as one resulting from a liberation of aggression.[c]

We shall not allow ourselves to be misled by the contrast between the comic and the sublime into forgetting that they serve a common purpose: *the mastery of an inner danger.*[d] (Italics mine.)

This function of laughter [superiority being a defense against anxiety] rests upon the formula: "I need not be afraid; it is laughable"—and . . . "I laugh, so I am not afraid, for he who laughs is powerful, strong and superior." . . . ultimately defense against anxiety, mastery of anxiety, and pleasure gain, are compressed together in the one act.[e]

This difficulty in drawing the boundary between humor and self-irony reminds us again how imperfect is any happiness which the comic can offer us. *We see man as an eternal pleasure-seeker walking on a narrow ledge above an abyss of fear.*[f] (Italics mine.)

Kris goes so far as to say that failure to find the sudden discomfiture of another person ludicrous* may signify excessive identification with him.[g]

Other contemporary Freudians share this view of laughter as an inadequate compensation for fearful or malign human tendencies:

The ostensible gaiety of laughter masks . . . fear, hate, madness, despair, regret, or triumph. Laughter results from a sudden reduction in sadistic psychic tensions.[h]

Comedy is a release of aggression. . . . The urge to tell a joke is

* Huckleberry Finn says of the laughter of the circus audience at the attempts of the supposedly drunken clown to mount a horse, "It wasn't funny to me . . . I was all of a tremble to see his danger."

> . . . a device for discharging of tensions of both . . . aggressions and guilt without . . . resolving the ambivalence.[a]

> Dreams with a manifest elated mood are well-known; dreams which contain laughter or which palm themselves off as "happy dreams" mean the reverse of what they seem to say. They contain latent death wishes or thoughts of one's own death.[b]

Edith Jacobson recognizes a wider range in varieties of laughter "from subtle tender amusement, on to bright and joyful, to mildly ironical, to grim sardonic or triumphant laughter"; but she stresses "laughing at another person's physical or moral failure . . . e.g., when a person stumbles and falls on the street." [c]

It is certainly true that one kind of laughter may be a defense against shame, as, also, against fear, self-distrust, anger, or aggression. The Gentleman in *King Lear* refers to:

> . . . the fool, who labours to outjest
> His heart-struck injuries.[d]

It also is true that great susceptibility to shame may lead a person to think that any laughter he hears is directed against him. Furthermore, it is sometimes possible to turn an experience from one of shame to one of humor by laughing at the grotesque inappropriateness of a situation in which one is oneself involved. By recognizing the ludicrous, laughing at it, one becomes the person who sees around oneself as an other.

But to assume that it is healthy or desirable to find the exposure of another person ludicrous, that it is a defect of identification if one does not, and that the chief source of laughter is a need to overcome fear of one's own exposure and to find pleasure at the discomfiture of another is surely to have an exceedingly meager theory of laughter, of humor, and of personality.* Repudiation of oneself as a human being as well as of the other person is involved if we find the exposure of another ludicrous. Moreover, humor according to this view is always interpersonal. It ignores the sense of the comic to be found in discrepancies in the nonpersonal world and in the relation of oneself and others

*See pp. 145-7 for other views of laughter.

to it. Of the whole theory of personality based on compensation for inadequacy or evil tendencies Kurt Goldstein says, "Freud fails to do justice to the positive aspects of life . . . even to the biological value of sex." [a]

Contemporary experimental psychologists and social scientists seem to have been more influenced by Freud's compensatory theory of personality than by his vast explorations into the unconscious. The conception of compensation in development of personality has been emphasized at the expense of other factors. Parsons and Shils say that conflict and anxiety are held "within the limits necessary for the working" of the personality system and that the failure of their smooth operation calls the special mechanism of defense and adjustment into play.[b] Dollard and Miller see the individual as "struggling in the grip of his social system" (whatever the particular social system may be), and infancy as "a period of transitory psychosis," when "the seemingly innocuous feeding situation can be fraught with emotional consequences," [c] presumably dire. Whiting and Child believe that the significant categories in which to classify the varieties of human behavior are "oral, anal, sexual, dependence, and aggression." [d] Robert R. Sears says that "the biological nature of man, coupled with his universal gregariousness, gives rise to various learning experiences that every child *endures* in one fashion or another." [e] (Italics mine.) Georg Simmel, like Freud, believed that antagonism is never absent from social relations and that hatred and a desire to dominate enter into all relations of intimacy.[f] Harold D. Lasswell stresses release of tension and compensation more than any positive purposes as motives for human action.

> . . . the tension between demands on the ego for both independence and dependence is intensified by a disciplinary-indulgent environment. This increases the likelihood of those *vigorous compensations against dependency* that enable many persons to impress upon others *their seeming courage, intensity of conviction and strength of will.*[g] (Italics mine.)

> . . . one of the principal functions of symbols of remote objects like nations and classes [is to serve] as targets for the relief of many of

the tensions which might discharge disastrously in face-to-face relations.[a]

In such accounts stress appears to fall on the extent to which action is an effort to get away from something rather than to go toward something, to compensate for a lack or an undesirable state rather than to seek to realize an aim. Certainly such compensatory motivation and behavior may be observed as characteristic of persons in our society, and may to some extent characterize all or most individuals in any conceivable society. But use of compensation as a general principle of explanation tends to crowd out attention to the dynamics of interest and purpose in personality development. Curiosity, thought, sympathy, tenderness, love, use of language and symbols, reaching toward other people, or exploring the world become in a compensatory theory mainly derived drives, sex-inhibited aims, quasi needs, or secondary processes. Tolman says of the whole human development of symbolism in language and literature that symbols are used "in default of" being able to present the actual symbolized object.[b]

Dorothy Lee summarizes this emphasis on compensation for lack to the exclusion of other dynamic factors in human development: "The premise that man acts so as to satisfy needs presupposes a negative conception of the good as amelioration or the correction of an undesirable state. According to this view, man acts to relieve tension; good is the removal of evil and welfare the correction of ills; satisfaction is the meeting of a need . . . peace is the resolution of conflict; fear of the supernatural or of adverse public opinion is the incentive to good conduct. . . ."[c] Lee would undoubtedly grant that explanations in terms of compensation account for some phases of development, more in some people and in some societies than in others, but she protests against the belief that compensation is the central factor in development.

Pleasure-Pain, Reward-Punishment Motives

Conceptions of psychological scarcity and of compensation as the chief dynamic in personality development lead to a restricted view of what Jeremy Bentham called the springs of action, what we now call motivation. Human possibilities are reduced to some version of a stimulus-response, pleasure-pain, reward-punishment system. Psychological and moral scarcity prevails in this psychic economy. Individuals seek pleasure or reward, or pleasure substitutes, and avoid pain or punishment. To each other, human beings become objects who are instruments for release of tension and who administer pleasure or pain, reward or punishment. "Under the term 'rewards and punishments' are included all the satisfactions and dissatisfactions which other people are capable of producing in a person." [a]

Hedonism, like pragmatism, can be stretched to account verbally for any human experience. But if it is so extended, either many of the most significant human experiences are actually omitted altogether, or distinctions among different kinds of experiences become so blurred that they are meaningless.

Freud himself speaks of two principles of mental functioning —the pleasure principle and the reality principle.[b] Both are variants of a compensatory theory of personality.

> [In the establishment of the reality principle] a momentary pleasure, uncertain in its results, is given us, but only in order to gain in the new way an assured pleasure coming later.[c]

Hartmann and Rapaport are at pains to make clear that the reality principle itself is a part of the pleasure principle, since, according to the Freudian theory of thought and ego development, adaptation to reality occurs because it is necessary to avoid pain and to secure a deferred or substitute pleasure. Hartmann says:

> Every progress of growth . . . can be viewed from the angle of changing of conditions under which adaptation takes place and of changing the methods used in complying with the demands of reality.[d]

> . . . the reality-principle is, in a sense, the pursuit of the pleasure-principle by other means.
>
> . . . In the development toward reality, the pleasure possibilities offered by the developing ego functions, *love and other rewards*

gained from the object, and at a later stage the gratification arising from the renunciation of instinctual satisfaction are all essential.[a] (Italics mine.)

In Freud's view other human beings are objects to be used instrumentally for release of tension, satisfaction of needs, and giving of pleasure.*

Freud considers it unhealthy that a sudden sexual approach by a man whom he pronounced prepossessing should not arouse erotic response in a girl of fourteen, completely without regard to her feeling for the individual making the approach. The idea that shame or sense of self-respect might have been involved seems not to have occurred to him.

I should without question consider a person hysterical in whom an occasion for sexual excitement elicited feelings that were preponderantly or exclusively unpleasurable.

. . . Instead of the genital sensation which would certainly have been felt by a healthy girl in such circumstances, Dora was overcome by the unpleasurable feeling . . . [of] disgust.[b]

Love "objects" in Freud's view are more or less interchangeable and should be easily replaceable one by another.

[After death] The testing of reality, having shown that the loved object no longer exists, requires forthwith that all the libido shall be withdrawn from its attachments to this object. Against this demand a struggle of course arises—it may be universally observed that man never willingly abandons a libido-position, *not even when a substitute is already beckoning to him.*

Why this process of carrying out the behest of reality bit by bit . . . should be so extraordinarily painful *is not at all easy to explain in terms of mental economics.* (Italics mine.)

[In mourning] the ego . . . is persuaded by the sum of its narcissistic satisfactions in being able to sever its attachment to the non-existent object.[c]

* Freud's use of the term object to apply to a human being who is a goal to satisfy a need is one example of the problem of distinguishing meanings from words presented by Freudian terminology in general. (See p. 88 n.) But the extent to which in his theory other persons are discussed in relation to an individual in terms of the ways in which they do or do not satisfy needs suggests that something more than the use of a word in a specialized sense is involved here. (Cf. Schachtel's discussion of the Freudian use of object in "The Development of Focal Attention," p. 317.)

[In melancholia] The result [of loss of a loved person is] not the normal one of withdrawal of the libido from this object and transference of it to a new one. . . .[a]

In *Civilization and Its Discontents* Freud summarizes and makes explicit the theory of psychological scarcity, the pleasure-pain theory of motivation, the threatening aspect of reality, and the resulting conflict between the individual and any possible society. Man strives for the twin objects of profit and pleasure.[b] The pleasure principle draws up the program of life's purposes, but it runs counter to the whole world, and the task of avoiding pain forces the seeking of pleasure into the background.[c] Voluntary loneliness and isolation from others is the readiest safeguard against the unhappiness that may arise out of human relations.[d] Religion, science, and art are sublimations of more primary impulses; art affects us as a mild narcotic.* [e]

The implications of Freud's view of the dominance of the pleasure-pain principle in human relations appear vividly in Proust's descriptions of the nature and limitations of love:

The lie as to what we are, whom we love, what we feel with regard to the person who loves us . . . that lie is one of the only things in the world that can open a window for us upon what is novel, unknown.[f]

Many contemporary Freudians maintain Freud's pleasure principle in its starkest form. Federn's "felicific calculus" is as much rooted in an economics of psychological scarcity and is as mechanical as Bentham's.

Two normal ways out of the mental pain from frustration follow the pain-pleasure principle. The first is to shift the libido, from the object which through frustration has become painful, to a new

* Herbert Marcuse extols Freud because Freud's insistence on the basic antagonism between individual impulses and social domination exposes the "spurious liberties, choices, and individualities" under which dehumanization and repression are in our present society concealed. But he translates Freud's biological determinism into historical processes. His conclusion that not any possible historical reality but this particular historical reality is hostile to man's desires may be justified in terms of historical analysis, not in terms of what Freud says. (*Eros and Civilization,* Beacon Press, 1955, pp. 99-100.) Cf. pp. 117, 153 n., 214.

object. The second is to occupy the mind with familiar objects which are known, either in reality or in fantasy, as pleasant. . . . Both pathways are identical psychodynamically; so far as the economic compensation is concerned, it makes no difference whether the libido investment is directed towards a new object or is added to that of an old one. There is a very exact economic proportion between mental pain and its compensations. The positive effect can be reached by a relatively small joy related to the object if that object was very important to the individual. . . . If only a small section of the ego is involved, the joy itself has to be greater.

Sadness is the painful ego state created by ceasing to love. If the love object was very important, the consequence of the loss quite frequently may be that love turns into hate. . . . This hate can give some satisfaction and diminish the sadness through the pleasure in seeking revenge. . . .[a]

Some contemporary psychologists, in attempting to effect a reconciliation between the experimental methods of Pavlov and Clark Hull in the study of motivation and the contributions of Freud, have tended to take over the most schematic and limited aspects of Freud's thought, those which challenge least and fit most easily into the experimental categories. They tend to use Freud somewhat selectively, and in so doing lose some of his most important insights. The reward-punishment, pleasure-pain concepts are not simply reflected in chance phrases, but form the almost unquestioned basis of much of their thinking.

Habit is a relationship between a stimulus and a response.[b] Parsons and Shils extend the definition of cathexis to include attachment to objects that are gratifying, rejection of those that are noxious,[c] a statement that can be read either as a platitude saying that energy reacts positively or negatively or, if it is more, brings all behavior into a pleasure-pain theory.

Most practices . . . lead to some kind of reward by other members of the society if properly* performed, or to some type of punishment if improperly performed.[d]

* It is not entirely clear what is included in "properly." It would seem to mean properly according to the codes of the society, rather than bringing in the possibility of any other standards and the kinds of questioning of the codes of the society that may be involved in deviant behavior or in shame.

Dollard and Miller prefer the term reinforcement to reward or the pleasure principle,[a] but the pleasure-pain principle is essentially unaltered:

> . . . all habits seem to obey exactly the same laws, e.g., the gradient of reinforcement, generalization, extinction, spontaneous recovery, etc.[b]

> As long as an individual is being rewarded for what he is doing, he will learn these particular responses more thoroughly, but he may not learn anything new by trial and error.[c]

> The goal of the whole therapeutic situation is to resolve the neurotic conflict and to set in place of it a positive, drive-reducing habit.[d]

Other learning theories, also, vary the statements and the experimental evidence rather than the basic concepts.

> The truth of the matter seems to be that all learning presupposes (1) an increase of motivation (striving) and (2) a decrease of motivation (success) and that the essential features of the process are much the same, regardless of the specific source of motivation or the particular circumstances of its elimination.[e]

Like psychologists, social scientists influenced by Freud have frequently taken over the most easily transferable features of his theory, to the neglect of its more complex and difficult dynamic aspects. In so doing they have actually violated the central animus of Freud's thought by aiming at logical completeness rather than continuing the slower and more difficult empirical study of genetic and dynamic processes.

This, for example, is Lasswell's scheme for comprehending all possibilities in human relations:

> Interpersonal relationships are *indulgent* or *deprivational*—or indifferent. . . .
>
> It is evident that the acts of a personality or a culture in relation to its interpersonal environment are also indulgent or deprivational—indulgent when they increase the deference, income and safety of the other personality or culture, and deprivational when they diminish deference, income and safety.[f]

Human beings behave on the basis of expected net indulgences over deprivations, unconscious as well as conscious.[a]

Here, in a system of analysis that aims to be logically comprehensive in regard to human behavior, mutual love and mutual discovery between human beings are ignored; values other than deference, income, and safety are ignored; working for the sake of enjoyment of good activity or for ends beyond one's own desires is ignored.

Such oversimplification of the range of desires and motives within the individual, and of the range of possibilities in relations among persons, may lead also to an oversimplified view of what is socially possible and socially desirable. What makes for relative simplicity and control in the study of the individual and of society may sometimes, subtly and unintentionally, become the criterion for what is desirable for the individual and for society.

This appears, for example, in the connotations acquired by such a word as hierarchy as applied to the individual and to society. Like the word primary,* hierarchy can carry the implications of a number of different meanings that are not always carefully differentiated from each other. The term hierarchy sometimes refers to time sequence—that which is first in the hierarchy is first in time; sometimes to relative strength; sometimes to relative predictive value. It is easy to see how reference to a hierarchy of needs in the individual or to a hierarchy of roles in society[b] may sometimes carry over (in the mind of the reader even without the intention of the writer) to the conception of first in the hierarchy meaning first in importance, or that to which most attention should be given, or even to that which is most desirable.

Dollard and Miller may be interpreted as meaning that only those persons described by Rorschach as extratensive,[c] who tend to live in terms of internal and external hierarchy, are normal: "Normal people have little motivation to talk frankly and extensively about their most significant problems." [d] They speak of an initial hierarchy of responses and of a new hierarchy

* See p. 87 for the different uses of the term primary.

produced by learning,[a] and of successive levels of adjustment.[b] They lay stress on "primary" functions of self-preservation and need in the individual, and on pride, power, and success in social relations. Such formulations, as noted above, appear to emphasize desire for security at the expense of discovery and new experience, for prestige at the expense of love and mutuality. Imagination seems paralyzed at finding other terms in which to describe the human enterprise, and analyses of personality and culture repeatedly revert to these terms.

This reward-and-punishment analysis of motivation may even carry over into what looks like manipulation of other persons for ends assumed by the social scientist, the psychologist, the teacher, or the therapist to be desirable. The term learning, much used by schools of thought that stress pleasure-pain, reward-punishment motivations, would seem to open out possibilities for growth, and to suggest awareness of and respect for the identity of other human beings. But to an observer, learning often seems to mean teaching, and teaching to mean manipulation. The social scientist, the teacher, or the psychoanalyst knows the correct answers. He is a clever manipulator of the citizen, the student, or the patient in terms of reward and punishment so that the subject of manipulation arrives at these correct answers. "The therapist must keep the balance of rewards for listening and rehearsing stronger than the punishments inflicted by rehearsal. . . . By teaching new verbal units we mean that the patient acquires [constructive] responses and that they are attached to the correct cues." [c]

Criticism by some contemporary psychologists of the attempts to compress human nature into this pleasure-pain, reward-punishment mold will be discussed later. Reward-punishment theories built on a model of psychological and moral scarcity make impossible the understanding of some of the deepest personal experiences, such as shame, identity, independent thought, and perception of and sense of moral values beyond those of a given culture. The inadequacy of such a model for human understanding is coming increasingly to be recognized.

But no more searching criticism has been made of the limitations of the reward-punishment explanation of human nature than John Stuart Mill's comment on Jeremy Bentham, early nineteenth-century exponent of the pleasure principle:

> [Bentham's] general conception of human nature and life, furnished him with an unusually slender stock of premises.
>
> . . . [He wantonly dismissed as] 'vague generalities' the whole unanalysed experience of the human race.
>
> . . . the faculty by which one mind . . . throws itself into the feelings [of a mind different from itself] was denied him by his deficiency of Imagination. Self-consciousness, that daemon of . . . men of genius . . . never was awakened in him. . . . He . . . recognized no diversities of character but such as he who runs may read.
>
> . . . his recognition does not extend to the more complex forms of [sympathy]—the love of loving . . . or of objects of admiration and reverence.[a]
>
> . . . Man is never recognized by him as a being capable . . . of desiring, for its own sake, the conformity of his own character to his standard of excellence, without hope of good or fear of evil from other source than his own inward consciousness.
>
> The sense of honour and personal dignity—that feeling of personal exaltation and degradation which acts independently of other people's opinion, or even in defiance of it; the love of beauty, the passion of the artist . . . the love of power, not in the limited form of power over other human beings, but . . . the power of making our volitions effectual . . . the thirst for movement and activity . . . None of these powerful constituents of human nature are thought worthy of a place among the Springs of Action.[b]

Mill was not unaware of the importance of the pleasure-pain principle in determining human behavior. There is no question that seeking of pleasure and avoidance of pain, even in their simplest form, do enter strongly into the processes of development. A scarcity theory of psychic energy, a compensatory theory of growth, and a reward-punishment theory of motivation do describe accurately and with penetration and clarity important aspects of human growth. It is when any of these, or all combined, are taken as exclusive principles of explanation that they are insufficient. These theories make reward and punishment too external to the experience itself; the "rewards" of mutual love, of scientific discovery, of artistic creation lie within the experience, not only in outside recognition of it. Pleasure-pain, reward-punishment theories used exclusively leave unexplained wide ranges of human feeling, thought, and action.

Neglect of History

Contemporary thinking in psychology and social science tends to work with little consideration of a time dimension, to take for granted, or to work within, the present structure and functioning of society. Psychologists and social scientists might be significantly divided into two groups according to whether they do or do not take historical change seriously into account in their thinking; whether they regard it as necessary to consider the particular historical setting of any phenomena they describe; whether they consider observed frustrations in human beings as products of an unalterable conflict between human nature and social reality or as products of specific social conditions that are inevitably changing in ways that can be, at least to some extent, influenced by men.

In the study of individuals, due in no small part to Freud's discoveries of the importance of early childhood and genetic factors in personality development, it has become accepted practice to include time perspective, the life history of the individual, in order to understand present and future behavior.[a] To a limited extent this recognition of the necessity of including the temporal dimension in order to understand any single action has carried over to social science. Thirty years ago it would have been the exceptional anthropologist who observed the details of child care and puberty rites in primitive societies; today no competent anthropologist would neglect such observations.

But recognition of the necessity of including the time dimension does not appear to anything like the same extent in the study of social groups and of society as in the study of individual personality. When E. H. Carr says that modern man is, beyond all precedent, "history conscious" he is emphatically not describing the so-called behavioral sciences at present in the ascendant in this country.

Their nonhistorical, or even antihistorical, attitude is a natural outcome of the reaction against the oversimplified evolutionary schemes of the eighteenth and nineteenth centuries, as well as of the current emphasis on empiricism and operational methods. In the last century Frazer and Morgan in anthropology, Comte and Spencer in sociology, had overreached their data in positing uniform development of different peoples through the same successive stages. Hegel's comprehensive system included much more adequate historical data and more complexity of thought, but his idealistic scheme absorbed too completely his recognition of the material aspects of reality. Marx deliberately overemphasized material and economic factors in historical development in order to bring to the fore essentials that he believed had been neglected. But both Hegel and Marx worked with a tacit acceptance of a belief in progress that is no longer possible for us in their terms.

Nineteenth-century students of society had too swiftly jumped to conclusions about "laws" of historical development, based on assumptions that took for granted more than they knew. In part because of this, there has been a tendency among twentieth-century social scientists to take the attitude that historical data are unnecessary or positively misleading; and that, therefore, change over time may be minimized in any scientific study of society. Because in different fields it has been necessary to reject oversimplified, automatic schemes of historical development, there has been a tendency to throw out all hypotheses about change in time, to concentrate on what can be observed here and now, and what can be deduced from such observations.

Thus, Karl R. Popper regards as a false or misleading 'historicism" any attempt to frame hypotheses about sequences of historical change beyond those applicable to limited situations of social engineering. "Instead of learning from the falsity of predictions to modify our hypotheses or to revise our estimates of particular historical situations, the whole field of historical knowledge becomes suspect." [a]

In the behavioral sciences nonhistorical treatment supposedly leaves out nothing essential for scientific understanding, makes for elimination of error, and makes possible the maximum simplification. Parsons believes that the present state of our knowledge precludes the possibility of any theory of change of social systems and that, therefore, any theory of change "in the structure of social systems must . . . be a theory of particular sub-processes of change *within* such systems, not of over-all processes of change *of* the systems as systems." [b] Lewis Coser in his elaboration of Georg Simmel's analysis of social conflict points out that contemporary social scientists are much more concerned with social stability than with historical change; that Parsons, for example, is primarily interested in the conservation of existing structures* and regards the conflicts involved in historical changes as "dysfunctional" phenomena, social pathologies to be reduced and as far as possible eliminated. Coser believes that Parsons' interest in mental health is partly explained "by his concern with mechanisms of social control that minimize conflict, and by his conviction that psychoanalysts and other mental health specialists can play a significant role in reducing deviance." [c]

Theories of human nature based on assumptions of psychological and moral scarcity and of the tendency of the organism always to restore a previous equilibrium contribute to this antihistorical attitude. Dorothy Lee says that she knows of no society where human physical survival has been shown, rather than unquestioningly assumed by social scientists, to be the main purpose of life. She believes that the compensatory theory of personality leads to an excessive emphasis on adaptation to

* The last chapter of Parsons' *The Social System* (Free Press, 1951) is entitled "The Processes of Change in Social Systems," and here and elsewhere he is at pains to say that he is interested in change as well as in the maintenance of the existing order. But his belief that we lack at present the basis for any general theories concerning changes of social systems results in the concentration on changes within the systems and on the maintenance of equilibrium Coser describes.

the society and belief that the healthy or happy person is simply the well-adjusted person.[a] Hartmann, as noted above, extends Freud's theory of the libido to include more interest in the development of the ego in its relation to the environment, but his accounts of the healthy personality always end in emphasis on the necessity of adaptation to existing society.[b] Obviously some degree of adaptation and adjustment of the organism to its environment is necessary for survival. But the central place given to adaptation in much contemporary psychological thought would seem to exceed this minimum necessity. Rapaport in his discussion of ideas as safety valves of drive tension and in his whole theory of thought and of personality constantly stresses the tendency to replace energy-disequilibrium by a return to a state of rest.[c] Such analyses as these, and of Parsons and Lasswell, appear to concentrate on the tendency of both individual and social organism to maintain equilibrium at the expense of directing attention to the tendency to change and grow.

If we were to take at face value some of the statements about the tendency of a society always to avoid basic or violent change, always if disturbed to correct itself and seek a former stasis, we could find no explanation of the fact that the human race is not still living in caves, or that feudal society did change into industrial society.

The movement of cybernetics, or feedback, has had a twofold influence on the human sciences. On the one hand, it calls attention to the important self-adjustive capacities of the nervous system and of the human organism, thus contributing to the evidence that leads beyond a scarcity theory of personality.

> Today, we are coming to realize that the body is very far from a conservative system, and that its component parts work in an environment where the available power is much less limited than we have taken it to be.[d]

On the other hand, there is some attempt to use the findings of cybernetics to minimize or neglect the process of social change and implicitly to encourage social quiescence. Norbert Wiener himself resists this tendency and is opposed to applying the findings of cybernetics prematurely to the social scene.[a]

Some writers make explicit what they believe to be the responsibility of social scientists and psychologists to manipulate people to desired ends. Kenneth W. Spence criticizes field theory in psychology because it fails "to provide us with laws which will enable us to control and manipulate the behavior-determining psychological field." [b] Lasswell expresses this view of social change.

> The configurative method of political analysis consists in the use of concepts of *development* and *equilibrium,* and in the adoption of *contemplative* and *manipulative attitudes* toward political change.[c]

The concept of normality or adaptation in terms of which the individual is manipulated by the psychologist or psychoanalyst and citizens and social institutions are manipulated by the social scientist is a concept that is determined by the existing standards of the dominant group in present society.[d] ". . . concepts of normality have become the morality of the mental hygienists, who subserve a class function." [e]

If discouragement with too expansive and ill-founded schemes of historical development has tended to confine attention to the immediate present, the insufficiency of theories of adjustment in the face of an uncertain future may bring reconsideration of the importance of historical understanding. Recognition of the hazards of the future in a time of social change that includes the hydrogen bomb may lead to the realization that we can have no adequate understanding of even the present moment, or ability to predict its possible outcomes, without having understanding of its history.[f] When it is possible to act by rules, understanding of historical development can be more easily dispensed with. But when we find ourselves in situations that do not correspond to any known type, where they must be placed in a large framework and probabilities must be assessed, knowledge of history is indispensable. Concepts of historical necessity are both justified and indispensable if we regard them, not as the basis for prediction of specific events, but as setting limits to the range of possibilities. Within this range we can form some judgments as to which sequences of occurrences are more probable and which ones are less probable. An analysis such as Paul Baran's[a] of the possibilities and impossibilities in the relations between capitalist and underdeveloped countries, while one may differ with certain aspects of it, is of great value in reaffirming the possibility of bringing the resources of intelligence to bear upon understanding the processes of history. Such analyses help to counteract the tendency to seize upon errors in historical hypotheses, to abandon, as Baran says, the attempt to understand history, and to lapse into agnosticism and passivity.

The attempt of psychology and social science to exclude history in the interests of abstract method, logical completeness, and a timeless objectivity may result in missing the concrete realities that these disciplines are attempting to understand. "Objectivity which rests on the reduction of men to creatures alien to humanity is in truth but solipsism in a different guise. . . . Attempted exclusion is unwitting inclusion, and involves at best self-deception and at worst a misleading of others." [b]

If, however, the psychologist or the social scientist does attempt to see his own particular problems of study in the full concreteness of their historical setting he cannot expect to find historical facts, periods, and sequences "as they really are," as Ranke hoped in the early nineteenth century. This does not mean, as is sometimes alleged, that history is an art as opposed to being a science, or that history deals with individual happenings in contrast to science, which deals with laws. What it does mean is that the historian, like the psychologist, the social scientist, or any other student, must recognize that facts do not "speak for themselves." No history is the whole of the time it recounts, and historical data do come ready-made, selected, and classified. The historian inevitably selects the problems and the data that seem to him most significant and classifies them in the way that seems most significant. His conception of what is important reflects the concerns of his particular environment, his class, and his own period of history.

Recognition of the particular interests and assumptions that the historian brings to his investigation is an aid, not a hindrance, to objectivity.[a] Denial of assumptions and of the values inherent in them does not eliminate the assumptions; rather, it obscures them so that they can be less easily examined and tested. There is no greater obstacle to the attainment of objectivity than mistaking awareness of the orientation of the observer for subjectivity.

This view of objectivity as including awareness of what the observer brings to his observations is part of a long and honorable tradition, although it has often been obscured by a limited view of scientific method. Goethe always rejected the idea that objectivity consists simply in excluding subjectivity and that the scientist can and must "eliminate himself and operate as it were *in absentia,* leaving his personality outside in the lobby like a hat or an umbrella." [b] Erikson in comparing Freud with Darwin speaks of "that dogged, that prejudiced persistence which is one condition for an original mind becoming a creative one." [c] Recently there has been greater recognition of the care needed to make sure that a scientific presupposition is not translated into a definition of what was to be proved, and of the extent to which the method used affects the data selected and the results obtained. Contemporary studies of perception describe perception as a process of interaction between the perceiver and the outer world.* The greater the awareness of the order inherent in the method of observation, the greater can be the knowledge of order inherent in the external world.[d] The more careful the definition of what the observer brings to the process, the greater the certainty of what is *there* in the outer world.

The necessity to define precisely his own assumptions and the boundaries of his observations is thus no special obligation laid upon the historian. The natural scientist must always make clear the basis of selection of his problem and data, the limits of the situation under study, and his tools of inquiry—all of which determine the scope and form, and to some extent the results, of his investigation. Even physics has to take into ac-

* See pp. 138-40 for discussion of the work of Schilder, Goldstein, Schachtel, and of Rudolf Arnheim and other Gestalt psychologists on perception.

count the effect of the instrument of measurement on the phenomenon measured.

The determination of what area or system or frame of reference we select as a basis for any historical study is a difficult one. But this difficulty we cannot evade. We cannot escape the choice between recognition of the particular frame of reference to which the historical processes under study are related and the illusion that we alone can transcend the limitations of our own historical situation. Objectivity is to be sought, not through a studied indifference to meanings, but through a heightened awareness of the assumptions used and values involved, making them clear and open to examination.

Some evidence of emerging interest in the time dimension in human affairs, even among the behavioral scientists, will be discussed later. There is beginning to be recognition that the choice does not lie between oversimplified, monistic theories of historical development and the rejection as useless of all attempts to discover meaning in history. Furthermore, there is beginning to be some awareness that even the prediction that is the core of operationalism cannot be engaged in without taking into account possible and probable sequences in historical development, limits set and options open.

Nothing-but Explanations

Through all the ways of phrasing the phenomena of personality and society that have been mentioned runs reductionism, the tendency to think that understanding results from reducing complex phenomena to their simplest elements, or to a single basic principle of explanation. Wholes tend to be reduced to parts, qualitative or organizational descriptions to quantitative statements, human strivings to compensations for frustrated primary needs, human development to response to reward and punishment, human relations to need-satisfying human objects, human society to its here-and-now, history-free structure and function.

"Surplus meaning" must be eliminated in favor of concepts more closely tied to the data,[a] and the data must be reduced to "nothing more" than certain stated empirical observations, which "completely delimit" the phenomena under study.[a] Such explanations are indispensable and illuminating for certain kinds of understanding and for understanding certain kinds of phenomena. Phenomena such as shame and identity they may miss, and as exclusive principles of explanation they fall short. As noted earlier, the effort to achieve what seems to be logical completeness, valuable as it is for some purposes, may lead to neglect of the full subtleties and complexities of important experiences. David C. McClelland briskly provides answers to a problem that has been of profound concern to philosophers from Socrates to Jean-Paul Sartre: "We have then four solutions to the conflict between excessive individualism and the need for solidarity; romantic love, individualistic striving for money or prestige, the unreal Kingdom of God on earth, and individualistic striving for service to others." [b] Talcott Parsons classifies the religious experience of mankind as a form of "non-empirical reality systems." [c]

Ruth Munroe, who describes herself as primarily Freudian in her orientation, believes that, although there are important aspects of personality that Freudian libido theory omits or slights, Freud cannot correctly be described as essentially "reductionist" in his thinking. The experiences that she cites as having "non-sexual" aspects[d] slighted in Freudian theory include: parent-child relations in other than their sexual aspects,[e] the child's inborn need for stimulus as well as for relief from stimulation,[f] the social situation of the child,[g] the need for security and self-esteem,[h] repercussions of group membership on behavior,[i] the self,[j] the self-image,[k] as well as, by implication, language, symbolism, scientific discovery and artistic creation.[l] Munroe notes that Freudian theory holds that man's inborn nature consists primarily of instinctual drives; that these drives are basically blindly sexual and blindly aggressive; that sexual drives are controlled mainly by anxiety; that Freud confuses acts that result in harm to persons or property with an inborn need to destroy;[m] that for Freud inanimate objects or ideas (the whole nonpersonal world of reality) are derivatives or substitutes;[n] that ego devices "which approach the normal" are still called "defenses."[a] She criticizes Freudian theory where it does show reductionist tendencies and urges that more attention be given to those aspects of personality neglected in Freudian thought. But she regards the omissions as correctable in terms of Freud's own theory, and she agrees with Marcuse in thinking that Freudian theory allows for much more expansion and richness in the interpretation of personality than the theories of his revisionist critics. She believes that the omissions are less significant than the range and multidimensional character of Freud's interpretations.

I think that Munroe underestimates the importance of the aspects of personality neglected in Freudian theory. They are important, I believe, because of the way in which the fact of these omissions has affected and continues to affect the central body of Freudian thought and the way in which it has been interpreted. But it is abundantly true that Freud's emphasis on overdeterminism or multiple causation in the *Interpretation of Dreams* and his dynamic interpretation of his clinical observations—"So varied in his grandiose one-sidedness," in Erikson's words—points the way toward more complex theories and richer individual and social possibilities than his stated conclusions would indicate.

"Freud makes it quite clear," says Schachtel, "that secondary process thought 'merely represents a roundabout way to wish fulfilment' . . . and that 'thinking is nothing but a substitute for the hallucinatory wish.' "[b] "The 'nothing but' view of man permeates Freud's work. It underlies the theory of the pleasure principle as well as that of the death instinct, just as it underlies the libido theory, the concept of sublimation, and the theory of thought as being nothing but a detour toward instinctual need gratification."[c]

Both Schachtel and Lionel Trilling, however, while stressing Freud's reductionist emphasis on the creative powers of man as substitute gratifications, recognize that Freud's great discoveries opened up possibilities for human development and creative achievement beyond what Freud himself envisaged. Schachtel points to the irony of the fact that the discoverer of a method of therapy that has done more than any other yet known to free man from bondage to his biological and individual past should himself have turned his eyes more in the direction of the inevitable tragedies rather than of the creative powers of life.[a] Trilling believes that Freud's hedonistic view of art cuts him off from any conception of what artistic meaning is. But, in spite of this, he sees Freudian psychology as the only psychology that takes full account of the dignity and tragic destiny of man, and which makes "poetry indigenous to the very constitution of the mind." [b] Thus what Freud has made possible in the content of art and poetry far outweighs the limitations he states as to their nature and origin.

The ignoring of the necessity of historical analysis for understanding human behavior, and of the extent to which what we call human nature is the product of a concrete historical situation, discussed above, is one more example of the fallacy of reductionism, a nothing-but way of thinking. Freud himself, well-versed as he was in the literature and mythology of other cultures, did not consider it necessary to study the history of Western European civilization or to consider social and economic differences between Western Europe and other societies in developing his theories of personality. He generalized from the historical period and the society that he knew.

Non-Freudian psychologists and social scientists have tended to work in terms of these limitations instead of following the implications of Freud's genius in clinical observations, his bold insights, and the dynamic and multidimensional qualities inherent in his theoretical statements. Marcuse, I believe, stretches Freudian theory too far in order to make his own criticism of our present performance-oriented society;[c] but his is the great virtue of having gone further than most other interpreters of Freud in seeing the heroic dimensions and revolutionary possibilities implicit in Freud's stated theories.

Contemporary Views of Language

Difficulty in communication was mentioned as a central characteristic of experiences of shame. Two major contemporary trends in the uses of language affect the possibility of communicating shame and similar experiences. One is a phase of reductionism. It is the endeavor to develop a fixed, unequivocal language of signs that eliminates ambiguity and surplus meaning. Bertrand Russell's ideal, for example, was a context-free language, like scientific language, in which there are absolutely simple particulars in the meaning of a word and in the thing designated by it.[a] The other is the attempt, derived from many sources and expressed in many ways, to enlarge the human capacity for creating and using symbols.

The emphasis on a language of signs or signals is a natural outcome of a number of contemporary trends: the need to find means of communication among peoples accessible to each other through mechanical means of communication but widely separate in culture, tradition, and habits of thought;[b] the faith in natural science and especially in positivistic science;* the anxieties and uncertainties that have led to protection by depersonalization.†

There is a natural tendency to feel that a kind of security would be offered by a language of signs whose meaning did not alter. For some persons processes of changes in language constitute a special threat. Communication that includes free verbal play with its inevitable risks of misunderstanding is for such persons something to be feared. "For them the conception and sense of the world implies and depends on an exact definition of words. Without this armor of verbal specificity they can not feel secure in their beliefs. . . . The insecure neurotic shrinks from free word-play; he tries to manipulate words mechanically, like machinery. He fears the adventure of communication." [c] One of the outcomes of traumatic war experiences has been observed to be a distrust and devaluation of language.[d]

For some purposes a language of signs, codes or signals is indispensable. Stop and Go signs, other shorthands of speech, exact mathematical and scientific signs need to be unequivocal

* Also called scientific empiricism and deriving in part from logical positivism.

† See pp. 184-95.

and invariable in meaning.* Western science has developed in part through the elaboration of such a language of signs. The language of signs makes possible scientific exchange among peoples where communication through any other means seems initially to be almost impossible. All language becomes a kind of code. George Herbert Mead believed that it is crucial for the development of a sense of self that one be able to communicate with others through words that have identical meanings for speaker and hearer.[a]

No one would question the importance, for various uses, of the elaboration of different forms of sign, code, and signal language. It is when an attempt is made to absorb all language into sign language, and when the distinction between sign and symbol is lost, that questions arise. An emotional response or a diffused experience such as shame may be dwarfed or falsified if it is too early or too exclusively confined to a particular label or category.

In much contemporary writing the distinction between signs and symbols is ignored. Of this tendency Cassirer says:

> Symbols . . . cannot be reduced to mere signals. Signals [signs] and symbols belong to two different universes of discourse: a signal is a part of the physical world of being; a symbol is a part of the human world of meaning.[b]

Symbols are treated as if they were signs. Symbolic logic uses the term symbol to mean sign. Joshua Whatmough elaborates with somewhat different emphasis distinctions in language between sign and symbols.†

Jung's rich study of symbols has been neglected not only by nonanalytical psychologists but by other schools of psychoanalysis. Therese Benedek remarks that speech is an "intellectual

* It has been pointed out that some of the signs used in psychology and social science are not as precise as they strive or appear to be. The terms pain and pleasure, reward, punishment, and reinforcement, widely used in describing the behavior in learning of rats and human beings, of children and adults, are not exact, precise terms.

†See pp. 171-81 for discussion of the meaning and uses of symbols and of Whatmough's views.

accomplishment" that is "not usually discussed in personality development."[a] Kubie traces all language development to bodily tension and the "symbolic" representation of the body.[b] Many academic psychologists tend to follow a particularly limited form of what is miscalled "symbolic logic."

It is because of its social origin that language and its derivatives, such as mathematics, are the most highly developed form of human *cue-producing* response.[c] (Italics mine.)

So much emphasis may be placed upon easy and obvious communication that experiences that are not readily communicated are ignored. From some psychologists recognition of nonfactual use of language comes as a concession; and the fact that it has to be mentioned emphasizes the fact that it is a concession. Thouless quotes:

> That thou, light-wingèd Dryad of the trees,
> In some melodious plot
> Of beechen green, and shadows numberless,
> Singest of summer in full-throated ease.

He comments, "It would be absurd to object to the use of language here that it conveys the minimum of factual information and that its choice of words and phrases is primarily determined by their affective meanings."[d] For Tolman language is an inferior substitute used "in default of" being able to present the actual symbolized object.[e] The logical outcome of this would seem to be to follow as far as possible Swift's recommendation: "Since words are only names for *things* it would be more convenient for all men to carry about with them such things as were necessary to express the particular business they are to discourse on."

There are obvious advantages for certain kinds of scientific precision of a language that concentrates on a limited exactness which demands elimination of ambiguity and complexity. The danger is that such concentration may mean impoverishment of other aspects and uses of language. Impoverishment of language has occurred before. In eighteenth-century France the effort to be scientific, combined with limited aristocratic usage, succeeded by the end of the century in reducing by almost two-thirds the rich vocabulary of the sixteenth century.[a] A language that is confined to labeling rather than defining, to denotation at the expense of connotation, does not have the means of expressing experiences whose nature includes ambiguity and surplus meaning. It omits from its purview some of the most significant dimensions of human nature, and possibly distorts others that it may seem to express more fully.

Limited exactness and the elimination of ambiguity in the use of language express the reductionist, nothing-but tendencies that run through the aspects of contemporary study discussed in this chapter. Necessary as such use of language is for certain purposes, it does not allow verbal expression of pervasive experiences such as shame and the sense of identity, and thus tends to constrict understanding of them.

FOUR

Emerging Ways of Studying Personality

This chapter will examine certain other approaches to the study of personality that, I believe, offer promise of greater insight into the elusive experiences of shame and identity. These emerging ways of studying personality are less generally used than those just discussed, but are beginning to gain recognition.

No other interpretations of personality, as far as I know, offer as clear and coherent a theoretical structure as those that rest upon such assumptions and work within such limits as those mentioned in the last chapter. Rapaport pays glowing tribute to the range and originality of Paul Schilder's contribution to the understanding of human personality:

> . . . there is hardly any area of psychiatric and psychological problems which Schilder did not recognize, tackle, and illuminate . . . hardly a [function] . . . which he did not explore . . . varieties of conscious experience, psychosomatic relationships, neuro-psychological inter-relations, epistemological foundations of our relation to reality, or the nature of man's socialization. . . .[a]

But he goes on to say that Schilder paid dearly for his encyclopedic mind in that he never rounded out systematically any of the infinitely rich observations and countless hypotheses he threw out in well-nigh all fields of psychiatric interest.[b]

Although probably none of the other persons mentioned in

this chapter has Schilder's range of interest and competence, Rapaport's comments on Schilder in some sense apply to them all. They are explorers more than they are makers of systems. Freud, too, was primarily an explorer and a creator of brilliant hypotheses, more interested in the implications of empirical observations than in the logical completeness of a system.[a]

New directions of attention in research, alternate interpretations of existing data, search for new models, do not lead immediately to new or proved systematic formulations, but they may point the way toward an enlargement of earlier conceptions. Again it must be emphasized that the various approaches to the study of personality suggested here are not alternatives but possible supplements or amplifications of those discussed earlier. Each cluster of ways of studying personality is in some measure dependent on the other for clues, hypotheses, suggestions for areas to be studied, and for methods of investigation.

Freud, in spite of the limitations of some of his emphases on separate subsystems within the personality, and on society as a shadowy, overgeneralized "reality," enriched, as no other single person has, the way in which personality is conceived. Adler and Jung brought into focus still other aspects of personality. The experimentalists, particularly in their study of certain conditions of learning, whatever the limitations of these studies, have added to our understanding. Behavioral social scientists, although they tend to minimize the importance of historical change, have contributed to our knowledge of concrete historical situations. The emerging conceptions discussed here do not mean a repudiation of the work of any of these individuals or schools of thought any more than Nils Bohr's work was a repudiation of Newton's. Earlier formulations are often not replaced but acquire new aspects when placed within a more general theory or one with different emphases.[b]

Some of the leading exponents of the methods described in the last chapter recognize the value of the newer insights. Melvin H. Marx states clearly that both constructive and reductive explanations are essential and that field theory should be welcomed as supplementing, rather than condemned as replacing, stimulus-response theory.[c] It is characteristic notably of

Freud, but also of some contemporary experimental psychologists, that the fullness and thrust of their observations tend to break down the more limited categories within which they have confined them. The contrast between the tough-minded scientists and the tender-minded philosophers no longer seems to hold.[a]

Small differences in direction of attention and in emphasis can, however, produce great differences in resulting interpretations, and these merit serious attention. There is coming into the open an active questioning of some accepted psychological axioms, assumptions, and idioms, and an attempt to seek more flexible and comprehensive theories. These are more than contradictions or refutations of earlier theories, or alternate positions on the same postulates; they are new organizations that change the *Gestalt*. Because of the difference in emphasis, some of the points combined in the preceding section are mentioned separately here because of their special importance.

Just because it is in the nature of these emerging ideas that they cannot be stated with the kind of precision to which we are accustomed, we must be careful not to dismiss them as imprecise, "fuzzy," or as an "anything is everything" approach. Some phases of investigation call for emphasis on small-scale precision, unambiguous clarity, and careful checking of minute detail—"tight thinking." In other phases if precision in small detail is made the criterion of validity it may impede understanding; "loose thinking" is necessary.[b] One phase, and one kind of thinking, is as necessary as the other. In an effort to establish themselves as sciences, psychology, early psychoanalysis, and in some areas the social sciences have emphasized tight thinking, analogies from the physical sciences, unambiguous data, and methods of minute precision. It is possible that at present certain kinds of understanding can come about only through the risks involved in "loose thinking." But we must bear in mind that the methods used and the concepts developed as described in this chapter were not arrived at in any effort to avoid the rigors of systematic analysis but through the necessity of following the implications of empirical evidence that would not permit of explanation in more confined terms. Some phenomena can be more truly described in larger and more flexible terms than in more minute and unyielding ones. Shame and the sense of identity are among the phenomena that must be reached in part through such methods.

No such statement of principles or assumptions in any field is ever final. The recurrent questions persist: How can we know? Where shall we begin? What boundaries shall we draw in a particular investigation? According to what categories shall we sort our data? What shall we regard as central? What analogies and metaphors shall we use in giving an account of the evidence? We never have definitive answers to such basic questions. We discover more fruitful ways of formulating them. These concepts, which are beginning to come into more general use, are, like all others, approximations in the light of our present knowledge and our history up to this point.

Search for Significant Wholes

Instead of making the criterion of validity the identification of isolable, unambiguous items of behavior that can be reduced to nothing-but statements devoid of surplus meaning, more effort is turned toward the discovery of significant wholes.

The discoveries of quantum physics have shown that the physical world cannot be understood through endless subdivision, and that the motion of a single particle cannot be understood except in relation to others. There can be statistical predictions about the behavior of a group of these phenomena, but not about a single one.*

Biology has always inevitably worked with the concept of organism. But recent biology has put less emphasis on atomistic (analytical and summative) descriptions of phenomena and more on the functioning whole. Analysis of individual parts of the organism is necessary, but is not enough, because each

* The implication of these references to changes in the physical sciences is not that psychology should seek to model itself on a new natural science, as it sought to model itself on an earlier one. But, when psychology does use analogies from natural science to suggest fresh ways of looking at its own data, the analogies should be drawn from present, not past, natural science.

individual part and event depends on the conditions within the whole; the actual whole exhibits properties not shown by individual parts, a principle of organization particularly characteristic of living systems.[a]

In psychology the work of Kurt Lewin, Max Wertheimer, Rudolf Arnheim,* and other Gestalt psychologists has been influential in directing attention to phenomena that can be understood only in relation to other phenomena as parts of larger wholes or fields.[b] Psychoanalytic psychology has not been uninfluenced by this *Gestalt* emphasis. Hartmann says that the assumption of an independent instinct of self-preservation has been replaced by the recognition that all available human equipment is co-ordinated in physiological and psychological processes which insure survival.[c] Bronfenbrenner, trying to co-ordinate various theories, bases his theory of personality on the assumption that the most significant aspects of human behavior are not relatively simple phenomena susceptible to rigorous experimental control, but are complex, somewhat elusive, and multidimensional.[d] Moreover, the vocabulary of holism, or field theory, or "molar" as contrasted with "molecular" terms has gained in popularity among psychologists.[e] Everyone agrees that the entire field or situation helps to determine the dynamics of the event, that for some purposes concentration on a relative whole, as for others concentration on a relative part, is necessary.

After all this has been said it is still true that long-ingrained habits of thought may still incline many students first to seek smaller units of study, then to relate them, and that much may be learned from a deliberate effort to consider larger units. It does make a difference whether there is first an attempt, partly unaware, to see into what irreducible parts a phenomenon may be broken down in order to get at the "real truth," or in

* "Shape and size of two units constantly define each other . . . any description of form in the static terms of sheer geometry, quantity, or location will fatally impoverish the facts . . . visual form is constantly endowed with striving and yielding, contraction and expansion, contrast and adaptation, attack and retreat [and so can] symbolize . . . action . . . by means of physically motionless objects." (Rudolf Arnheim, "Gestalt Psychology and Artistic Form," in Lancelot Law Whyte, *Aspects of Form,* Lund Humphries, 1951, p. 199.)

what significant relationships it must be considered in order to comprehend it.

This question remains: How shall we determine what is the most promising field, or significant whole, for a particular study? There is no more difficult question than this. But without the heightened awareness that the use of a field approach gives, the question may be overlooked or the answer taken for granted.

Any particular whole is no more a given than is any particular part. The atom is a whole in relation to its parts, a part in relation to the solar system. The child is a whole as compared with his cells or with his specific needs or wishes, a part as compared with his family, his play group, or the country. As we face in one direction we see smaller and smaller units, in the other increasingly larger ones. Consideration of the possibilities and limitations of selecting a particular system or whole as the significant field of study, not assuming it in advance, becomes part of the investigation for which we must take responsibility. ". . . a method of classification . . . that is based on the fundamental concept of 'being contained within' rather than of 'being separate from,' can . . . allow us to be sophisticated both about particulars and about wholes without falling into either meaningless particularism or vague and useless generality. It is simultaneously synthetic and analytic. . . . It rejects the dichotomies, the Aristotelian division . . . and yet furnishes us with a theoretically satisfactory principle of classification and analysis." [a]

In determining whether a larger field of relations or a smaller and possibly more isolable area is to be used in a particular investigation, both the nature of the particular phenomenon to be studied and the particular predisposition of the investigator must be taken into consideration. On the first, Konrad Z. Lorenz says:

> The research worker confronted with an organic system is under the methodological obligation to ascertain to what extent and in what regards [it] is a system of universal interaction and to what extent and in what regards it is a mosaic built up of unchangeable

and independent structures. . . . The biologist and particularly the behavior student must maintain an absolute readiness to use both methods; which of them has to be applied at a given moment is a question that . . . must be answered by patient inductive research, separately for each object and at every single step of the investigation.[a]

To the second applies all that has been said about the necessity of taking the presuppositions of the observer and his methods of observation into account in appraising his results.*

Facing in the direction of holism does not solve the questions of what the boundaries of a particular investigation should be or what the methods most suitable to it are. It does, however, force us to consider taking larger steps than are usually taken in an investigation, going beyond artificial "cut-off points" that sometimes lose precisely the unknown that is the object of search, and dissecting problems as needing investigation that have become so embedded in familiar ways of viewing data that they have come to be regarded as already solved.[b]

Freud, even with his concentration on specific biological needs rather than on specific social situations and his omission of reference to the self, did much to bring about this more inclusive approach to the understanding of personality. By bringing hitherto neglected aspects of personality into the area of serious study, by tracing the origins of adult behavior, by treating emotion and reason, sleeping and waking life, normal and abnormal behavior as a continuity, he, more than anyone else, brought into being a holistic view of personality.

No matter how great the contemporary stress on isolation of discrete units of study and minute precision of measurement, after Freud it is less possible to make these procedures a substitute for the knowledge of man. "This zeal for uncriticizable statements and precisely verifiable measurements should certainly be encouraged, but not without the warning that in pursuing Certainty, the Absolute, one is likely to leave Man,

* See pp. 112-14. Working with larger units has been more characteristic of sociologists and anthropologists than of psychologists because their area of interest almost by definition includes relations. It is more characteristic of anthropologists now than it was in the nineteenth century.

the thinking reed, forsaken in the rear. . . . 'You can't make a leaf grow by stretching it.' " [a]

Paul Schilder faced clearly toward holism. He believed that holism or field theory is not one more method to be added to an essentially segmented, lineal approach, but that all experiences can be understood only if they are studied in the setting of their relationships.

> We talk about aggression and submission, about activity and passivity, as if we were dealing with independent entities in the realm of the personality. . . . Aggressiveness and activity do not exist outside the situation in which they come into play. There is no instinct of aggressiveness. We should not talk about instincts, but about situations, and describe the situations and the actions necessitated by the situations. [There is a] deep inner relation of aggressive and destructive tendencies to investigation, trial and error.[b]

> There are no isolated experiences; every experience points to something else.[c]

> The simple reflex mechanisms are crystallizations of previous global and undifferentiated processes. So do habits automatize into relatively stable occasional apparatuses from undifferentiated and goal-seeking processes.[d]

Goldstein's work on the biology of the nervous system and on the behavior of brain-injured persons led him to the conclusion that neither the organism nor the personality can be understood by studying its parts in isolation and only then looking for a co-ordination of the whole, nor can even the parts themselves be accurately appraised in this way. It is the sick or damaged personality, he believes, whose relation to the world can most correctly be described in segmental, additive terms; nothing less than a holistic approach can accurately account for the behavior of the fully functioning person.

> A specific performance . . . is a specific pattern of the whole organism. . . . Each stimulation always causes a change in the entire condition, and only apparently a locally confined change.[e]

> The reaction to stimulation is always determined by the functional significance of the stimulus in that part of the organism

within reach of the stimulus. In the intact organism this reaction is determined by the whole; in the injured organism by the part which is relatively isolated.[a]

Goldstein's view does not deny that specific structures have special functions and significance, but it does deny that the functioning of any part of the organism can be understood by itself out of relation to the whole.[b]

The kind of emphasis that Goldstein and von Bertalanffy place on the functioning of the sensory-nervous system as a whole is a rejection of vitalism as well as of mechanism. Both mechanism and vitalism assume that the organism is a mechanistic sum of its parts, but vitalism adds the bringing in of an outside agency of control. A holistic view holds that the control, the life process, exists within the whole functioning organization of the parts.

Similar evidence of the necessity of understanding through relative wholes comes from the development of projective diagnostic tests. Hermann Rorschach repeatedly insisted that no part of the test that he created could be used as diagnostic apart from the rhythm and balance of the whole.[c] In an important series of papers Ernest Schachtel gives an exceptionally penetrating and imaginative analysis of the meaning of perception implicit in Rorschach's discoveries.[d] He develops the idea that perception cannot be understood as an isolable factor in personality but only as an aspect of the total personality, an aspect in which sensory experience, emotion, and intellect are all involved. He adds the important emphasis that perception is different in different historical epochs.[e]

Munroe, on the basis of teaching projective methods of testing, describes the difficulty of getting students who have been trained in a lineal codification of reality to develop awareness of more pervasive experiences. She believes that the insights of Jung can be of great importance in developing awareness of pervasive experiences.

I often feel that if [the students] had read Jung I would not have to struggle so hard to convey a sense of *underlying trends* revealed in the test materials instead of the direct *linkage* of test data with behavioral trait or identifiable instinctual drive, role, or diagnostic entity which students trained in academic psychology tend to expect.* [a]

Munroe comments on the difficulty of combining in a coherent theory of personality psychoanalytic theories of separate, distinct drives arising from internal stimuli and academic psychological theories of separate and distinct responses to external stimuli.[b]

Increasing attention to relative wholes has special relevance to the understanding of shame if I am at all right that a guilt-axis interpretation of personality tends to be atomistic, with emphasis on each separate act, with personality conceived as built by a series of additive steps, whereas a shame-axis interpretation is more related to the whole self.

A special phase of the increasing awareness of the importance of a holistic approach—namely, the emphasis on the self in contemporary psychological and psychoanalytic thought—is so central to the main problems raised in these pages that it will be discussed in a separate section of this chapter.

Study of Change and of the Apparently Trivial

Allied to field theory is the recognition of the importance of dynamic factors, that is, factors making for change, as essential to the understanding of any whole or field. The concept of process, referring to any changes occurring in a phenomenon or in a group of phenomena over a period of time, is becoming more important in the thinking of psychologists and social scientists. No one would deny that objects and events are subject to change in time, even those that seem most unchanging.† The question is how much and what kind of attention should be

* The idea of underlying trends is, of course, important in sociological and anthropological thought and in some schools of psychology apart from Jung. Even such a technique as "content analysis" includes "thematic analysis" as well as "item analysis."

† Cf. the statement that what are called structures in biology may be regarded as slow processes of long duration, what are called functions as more rapid processes of short duration.

given to change in time. Like the fact that the different phenomena under investigation affect each other, changes taking place in the objects under investigation constitute a difficulty for the investigator. But what does one do with this difficulty, which is also an inescapable and important aspect of the phenomena being studied? In striving for scientific exactness there has been some tendency to select areas for study affected as little as possible by change, or to study separate items or units of behavior *as if* they were unaffected by time, and only later to introduce the time factor. One of the emerging trends in the study of personality is the attempt to include in the investigation of any phenomena, change or process, and the dynamic factors involved in making a particular process what it is.

Here again there is no either-or. Some phenomena are less affected by changes in time than others, and even for those that are more affected it may be necessary for some purposes to study them in an abstract or artificial situation, ignoring the time factor. But keeping in mind that such study *is* an abstraction, not a description of the full concrete situation, is both important and difficult. This makes it the more necessary to recognize the effect of changes in time and to direct specific attention to them. The word process, made familiar by Alfred North Whitehead and John Dewey, among many others, is sometimes used as if it were self-explanatory, without clarification of the ways in which phenomena are understood differently by means of this concept. It can be simply a name attached to observations that remain essentially static. Taken seriously, however, it can become a way of opening up new problems, which drastically alters perception of phenomena and organization of experience.

The generation in which Freud grew up naturally, almost inevitably, framed theories in terms of the analogies of classical physics and an economics of scarcity. Neither type of analogy is any longer possible for us. Nor are the analogies based on the idea that evolution means inevitable progress. The age of quantum physics, of a potential economy of abundance, of spatial as well as global intracommunication has not found its appropriate analogies. Whatever these may be, we can be sure that they will include a complex, not a lineal, theory of causation,* some conception of inseparability of structure and function, of content and form, explanation in terms of organization of parts, and some concept of factors involved in change over time.

Plato sought truth by attempting to eliminate all changing, individualizing characteristics of observed phenomena, and thus to approach their reality, beyond change, beyond time and space, beyond all conditioning and qualifying factors. He attempted to arrive at knowledge of what a thing *is* by eliminating all possible conceptions of what it is *not*. When all layers of error had been peeled off, truth remained. Error and truth were polar opposites, incompatible with each other. All opposites for Plato were antitheses, polarities. Large is what it is because it is the antithesis of small; hard of soft; light of dark; day is the antithesis of night. There is no continuity or common ground between them. Opposites epitomize contrasts with each other. Aristotle made of this conception of opposites a logical theory of identity, nonidentity, and excluded middle. A is A. A is not not-A. X is either A or not-A.

Hegel sought truth by attempting to discover what a thing —an object, an idea, a belief, a historical period—*is,* or may become, in its fullest dimensions.[a] Instead of eliminating, he took everything in. Instead of trying to discover truth by peeling off layers of untruth, he attempted to discover the truth of any conception by acting upon its hypotheses as if it included all truth. Only when its full possibilities have been explored does it reveal its limitations; it is not all; there is more in the world; there is an other. This other, this more, is in one sense an opposite, but it is an opposite continuous with and growing out of the original conception, not postulated as being at the opposite pole from it. Thus, although the same term—opposite —is used in describing Plato's and Hegel's thought, the two

* Complexity as used here does not imply a contrast to certain kinds of simplicities as they are sought, for example, in Gestalt psychology. It implies, rather, a contrast to a kind of analysis that in the supposed interest of simplicity omits certain essential factors.

conceptions arise from an almost wholly different way of thinking.

For Hegel, taking anything in its full dimensions involved including its time dimension, understanding it as changing, for change is a characteristic of all things. Truth is to be found by including time, not by attempting to eliminate time. Attempting to isolate any phenomenon as static is to place it in an artificial, false position. Change is of the essence of reality. Hegel's philosophy is a development of the conception of process.

Kurt Lewin's dynamic theory of personality* makes distinctions, similar to those between Plato and Hegel, between a psychology rooted in Aristotelian physics and one rooted in Galilean and post-Galilean physics. Aristotelian thought makes use of classifications based on frequency of occurrence and on the ignoring of single occurrences and individual, "accidental" characteristics; makes use of products rather than processes; of paired Platonic opposites; of the concept of antithesis between scientific law and individuality; and of isolation of the phenomenon to be studied. In physics since Galileo, not only is nothing a priori trivial or unimportant, but dichotomous classifications have been replaced by concepts of continuous gradation. Phenomena can be understood only if they are seen as in "continuous variation," with transition stages always present.[a] Tracing the continuous changes that produce a particular result may be fully as important for understanding as the final outcome. "Impatience asks for the impossible, wants to reach the goal without the means of getting there. The length of the journey has to be borne with, for every moment is necessary." [b]

Developments of quantum physics have carried still further the concepts of the necessity of including time in the description of phenomena, of the possible importance of the seemingly trivial, and of description in terms, not of polarities or of dualities, but of continuous gradation. Instead of the atoms acted upon by forces of Freud's day, we have reality phrased in terms of interaction rather than separation, continuities rather than polarities, multiple possibilities rather than dualities,

* See pp. 127, 152 n., 168.

probabilities rather than precise prediction of a single event.[a]

Freud himself expressed his discoveries in terms of the physical and economic analogies of his time, but, as has been said repeatedly, his clinical observations and his stress on dynamic continuities carried the implications of his thought beyond his own theoretical categories. Recognition that there is nothing incidental or unimportant in human behavior, that the small, specific, individualizing details of an experience (the kind of trivial details that are at the heart of an experience of shame) may be of special importance, was one of Freud's great achievements. Memory in dreams, he observed, recalls not essential and important, but subordinate and disregarded things. The result of these observations and attempts at explanation had often, according to Freud, to be expressed in "nebulous, scarcely imaginable conceptions" which will be more clearly apprehended as the process of understanding continues.[b] Nothing can be ignored simply because it cannot be classified. Everything is a part of an ongoing process, and helps to make the process what it is.

Harry Stack Sullivan similarly stressed the importance of the apparently incidental. His observations led him to the conclusion that the significance of particular courses of events in personality development inheres in nuances more than in the gross pattern more easily put into words, and that awareness of the marginal processes of thought gives more insight than accounts of the more obvious experiences.[c]

Schilder, in his explorations of the dynamics of personality development, both questioned and carried forward Freud's theories. He gave great importance to an individual's awareness of his own body as an inescapable part of the life process. The kind of perception human beings have of their bodies, the image they hold of them, is peculiarly involved in shame. Certain features of one's own body are unalterable, uncontrollable; in a unique way, they are oneself. Sudden exposure of them (Dmitri's sudden awareness of the exposure of the shape of his toes, Philip's clubfoot, Levin's blushes), or lack of control of them (Lear's "hot tears, which break from me perforce"), or awareness of the difference between the way one sees his own body and the way others may see it—all these are experiences of shame deeply associated with the quick of oneself, with one's own identity. Schilder makes clear that, as in all perception, this inescapable intimacy with one's own body is a two-way interchange, an interaction of external and internal; tactile and other bodily impressions are shaped by contact with objects, as impressions of the external world are derived from bodily sensations. One experience is not possible without the other.[a]

Thus the body image is in part a social phenomenon. One's body image helps to shape one's image of the world, and one's image of the world affects the image one has of one's own body; both parts of the process are essential. Schilder believes that the conception of other persons as audience—so stressed in the usual definitions of shame—has been overemphasized, and that interest in exploring and adorning one's own body is as inborn as the desire to display it and to see the bodies of others. Because of this interest in one's own body there is concern about the integrity and beauty of all parts of the body, not only about the sexual organs. The "castration complex" is only one expression of the fear of dismemberment and the desire for integrity of all parts of the body. The loss of the sense of integrity of one's body and of intimacy with it results in a sense of depersonalization, loss of one's own identity, which is a symptom of mental disease.[b]

Central in Schilder's thinking is a dialectical concept of process, a concept of opposites as parts of a continuous gradation complementing and enlarging each other in Hegel's sense, not as mutually exclusive polarities in Plato's sense.

> There are no elements of sensation, feeling, imagination, and thinking. There are processes going on which bring the various aspects of the total situation into the foreground. . . .
>
> So-called stimuli are probably never merely internal or external. We react to the world according to the internal state in which we are. There is no purely internal state because we are always directed toward the world. Internal and external are correlated with each other.[c]

> . . . to think in polarities . . . is merely a habit without regard for the real structure of things, and excusable only as a preliminary

step in the explanation of the world. If one observes carefully enough, true opposites are not found. . . . Warm is not the opposite of cold. Dark is not the opposite of light, love is not the opposite of hatred. . . . There is no polarity between activity and passivity, between aggression and submission, between rest and motion. . . . I have never found two opposite strivings as the basis of so-called ambivalence . . . masculinity is not the opposite of femininity.[a]

Goldstein, like Schilder, believes that understanding is reached through the study of continuous change in whole organisms more than through attempted isolation of parts.

The customary method [of biology] attempts to "reduce" variable to constant reactions, seeing, in the latter, the basic ones, and regarding the former as modifications. . . . There is no justification for calling one the normal reflex, and the others variations of it. If one does think this way, he does so only under *the theoretical preconception which claims that a phenomenon is normal when found in the artificial isolation of an analytic experiment.*[b] (Italics mine.)

Consciousness of self and consciousness of objects are to him complementary experiences, essential to each other. In a catastrophic condition that makes ordered reactions impossible a person loses both any clear awareness of objects in the outer world and any clear awareness of himself. For the healthy person consciousness of objects and of himself increase concurrently.[c]

Rorschach's method of interpreting the test that he designed is a striking example of the use of continuity through change in time for the interpretation of personality. Underlying his whole method is the conception that style and organization are more basic than the specific content or quantitative distribution of experience. The emphasis is on how, and in what proportion and relation, rather than on how much.[d] Like Schilder, Rorschach believed in the sterility of concepts of opposites in the Platonic sense: "What appears clinically as antithesis, is, psychologically, simply variation"; it is not true that introversion and extroversion are really opposites.[e] He regarded the process of arriving at a particular perception as more significant than the end result reached; the contingencies and the kinds of possibilities that enter into reaching a conclusion are of more importance in revealing personality than the conclusion itself.[a]

The study of perception by Gestalt psychologists has done much to break down the dichotomy between inner and outer, subject and object, and to develop the idea of continuous gradations of change in the study of personality. But in the writings of Wolfgang Köhler, Wertheimer, and others it is not always entirely clear to what extent "order" lies within the perceiving self, or in the external world, or in "isomorphism," the correspondence between the structural organization of the perceiving self and the structural organization of the physical objects perceived.[b]

From a wealth of detailed observations, Schachtel has elaborated the view of perception, not as an isolated or detached part of the personality, nor as an area separate from the study of personality,* but as an expression of the whole personality,[c] and as a continuing process in which subject and object are both differentiated and related. He makes it clear that there is no such thing as objectivity into which the thoughts, feelings, and values of the perceiving self do not enter, and that more of the aims of objectivity are gained by recognizing the way in which the observer enters into observation than by assuming that he can be excluded.

What we perceive is determined to a considerable extent by what we are taught and accustomed to perceive, but also by what we wish and what we fear to perceive. Out of the infinite number and variety of visual stimuli surrounding man at any given moment and place, only a relatively small selection enters his actual perceptions.[d]

Mankind cannot transcend human thinking nor can the individual person transcend that way of thinking which his personal history together with his constitution have developed in him. . . .[e]

Either completely detached objective or completely subjective experience is an impossibility; every experience is a compound of both. Attempts to be detached result in both an enrichment and an impoverishment of perception.[f]

* Cf. p. 80.

[Focal attention develops from] a diffuse total awareness . . . in which at first there is no distinction between the infant and the environment . . . to . . . a state in which distinct needs and feelings become increasingly differentiated and discrete objects emerge from the environment. Ultimately, these objects are conceived by the child to have an existence of their own that continues even when the object does not impinge on the child's receptors.[a]

T. S. Eliot has reminded us that continuous interflowing of thought and feeling, of the perceiving self and the perceived world, has been experienced by some people as a reality in certain periods of history:

A thought to Donne was an experience [a direct sensuous apprehension]; it modified his sensibility. When a poet's mind is perfectly equipped for its work, it is constantly amalgamating disparate experience; the ordinary man's experience is chaotic, irregular, fragmentary. [He] falls in love, or reads Spinoza, and these two experiences have nothing to do with each other, or with the noise of the typewriter or the smell of cooking; in the mind of the poet these experiences are always forming new wholes.[b]

Donne's poetry . . . was born in part out of an increase in self-consciousness. . . . What he strove to devise was a medium of expression that would correspond to the felt intricacy of his existence. . . . Donne's technical discoveries did not belong to him alone. They were a product of a whole mode of thought and feeling . . . the richest and most varied that has ever come to expression in English . . . for all the most notable poets of Donne's time there was no separation between life and thought. . . . It was as true for these poets as for Donne that 'a thought was an experience' which modified their capacity of feeling.[c]

Such congruence of feeling and thought, subject and object, awareness of inner anticipations and memories that find their dialectical counterpart in the outer world of people and of things is the stuff from which a sense of identity is formed.

Amplification of Compensatory Theory

Such a conception of an active, reciprocal, developing relation between feeling and thought, subject and object, the individual and the outer world, leads beyond a compensatory theory of personality. Accurately as a theory of compensation accounts for many aspects of personality development, particularly in our contemporary society, there are other aspects that cannot be adequately accommodated within it.

Human beings, according to the theories of process just described, are seen to have capacities for being spontaneously active and creatively interested in other persons and in the nonpersonal world that find only meager expression in what we call human behavior or human nature in our society. In this perspective, goals, instead of being only specific objects to release tension, become expanding purposes in which the whole personality may be involved. Wonder, curiosity, interest, thought, sympathy, trust, love are seen as characteristic human attributes, not simply as secondary, derived aims. Reality becomes something capable of yielding knowledge, interest, and fulfillment instead of being mainly a threat to be coped with. A whole philosophy of society and of history is expressed in the widely current use of the phrase "coping with reality," which implies that society and reality are felt as difficulties or dangers by the individual, something to be warded off, coped with, or at great sacrifice adjusted to.* A psychology of potential abundance may replace a psychology based upon an economics of scarcity.

As in the use of the word process, the question must be raised whether introducing different terms alters ways of thinking and methods of investigation. If behavior is described as positive instead of negative, active instead of passive, self-actualizing

* Questioning of the conception of reality as something to be coped with does not imply that reality can ever exclude conflict or that conflict is necessarily "dysfunctional." It implies only that society and reality can be something other than threats to human beings.

instead of need driven, does this mark simply a verbal difference or is it an actual difference in conception which changes the way we see and study personality? Is anything gained by distinguishing between need and value, between barrier and goal, between superego and ego-ideal? [a] The question must also be raised whether in these different emphases we are simply indulging in wishful thinking, ignoring either inevitable human tragedy, or the inevitably repressive character of our own achievement, performance, success-oriented society.

I believe that the phrasing of the phenomena of personality development, not only in terms of compensation for frustration of specific needs, but in terms of directions of the whole self, can make a genuine difference in the kinds of questions to which attention is directed, the kinds of experiences considered important for study, the kinds of hypotheses entertained, the models and analogies considered appropriate, and the range of human variations and possibilities envisaged. It does make a difference whether the individual is considered as eager, curious, and trusting until specific experiences in a given society and historical period lead him to be anxious, cautious, and aggressive, or whether he is regarded as born with hostility, aggression, and fear which specific experiences may modify only to a limited degree in the direction of trust, sympathy, and interest. It does make a difference whether personality is conceived primarily in terms of an economics of psychic scarcity and threats to the self or whether every stage of development is regarded also as accompanied by greater resources of energy.[b] It also makes a difference whether the frustration of human possibilities is laid to relatively unchanging biological drives inevitably frustrated by any conceivable society or, at least in part, to the specific repressions in the particular historical societies we have known. If the first, it is useless for men to try to make a more humanly livable society; if the second, men can, at least within limits, make their own history.

Here again, the contrast can be overemphasized, and the implications of some of Freud's observations point toward wider interpretations than his own formulated conclusions.[c] But conceptions of a fund of inborn aggression and of any world of reality as a threat to individual desires did color Freud's own thinking, and have had an influence disproportionate to other parts of his theories on later Freudian thought and on non-Freudian psychology.

Henry A. Murray and Gordon Allport, among others, have repeatedly stressed the limitations of the models currently used in the study of personality and the highly selective and subjective picture of personality that emerges from such studies under the guise of scientific objectivity. Murray holds that insistence on the physiological animal analogy is one of the great obstacles to the understanding of human beings.

> One of the granite boulders of cognition, from my eccentric and unfashionable viewpoint, is the model of the culture-clear, conscience-free, maze-imprisoned, hunger-driven, cheese-seeking rat, which is forever engraved on the entablatures of our cortices.[a]

Allport says:

> If it is the child's nature to trust everyone, why is it the nature of national or ethnic groups to distrust nearly everyone? The models we have been following tend to deflect our attention from problems of human affection and the conditions for its development. When a bit of human friendliness is discovered—and it can be discovered only accidentally with models now current—it is likely to be labeled "goal-inhibited sexuality," and thus tagged, forgotten.[b]

More adequate models are yet to be conceived. As Murray has said, if the personality is treated *only* as a whole, and if all actions are attributed to one over-all drive—whether it be Freud's early conception of libido, Fromm's self-realization, or Goldstein's self-actualization—no action and no person can be distinguished in his motives from any other.[c] A self-actualizing view of personality still demands—what is sometimes ignored—the study of subsystems and their relation to each other. But if we view personality as active rather than as inert until stimulated,[d] if we accept the idea that human beings are concerned with something more than the satisfaction of specific needs and the return to a previously established equilibrium,[e] then we can begin to give serious study to what this something more is; we can inquire into the processes involved in attaining the new situations which differ from the previous state of rest and into the kinds of social conditions most favorable for human development.

Conceptions of abundance rather than scarcity of psychic energy appear even in psychoanalytic views regarded as orthodox. Franz Alexander asserts explicitly that "Erotic phenomena do not follow the principle of inertia. They are designed not to save energy but to spend it spontaneously. . . . The energy spent in this lavish experimental and playful manner is surplus energy, not used for preserving homeostatic stability or survival." [a]

Schilder affirms the view of personality as actively searching, and goes into some detail as to what this conception means and where it may lead.

> . . . human beings have a genuine interest in the world, in action and in experimentation. . . . They do not experience reality as a threat to existence . . . human organisms, have a genuine feeling of safety and security in this world. Threats come merely from specific situations and deprivations.[b]

> Actions are directed toward objects. . . . Identification is therefore not, as Freud states, the earliest and most original type of emotional cathexis. . . . Before the boy identifies himself with his father he has an interest in him.[c]

> Desires and instincts cannot be understood as mechanical agents. They have aims and purposes. . . . Drives and desires go beyond mere satisfaction. They do not tend simply to bring the individual back to a state of rest; they thrust outward towards the world. . . . It is Freud's basic assumption that desires intend to establish a state of rest. I think that this assumption is fundamentally wrong. . . . The world of Freud is a shadow world, as far as the individual is concerned.[d]

Goldstein goes even further. He says, not only that the basic, more generalized experiences are those of trust and interest in the world, with fear of the world and aggression developing later in response to specific social situations, but that when one reverses this sequence what is described is not personality, but sick personality. In his view the overriding necessity for release of tensions or satisfaction of specific needs is characteristic of the sick human being or of the laboratory animal, not of the healthy human adult. When fear, aggression, segmentation, necessity for release of tension or resolution of conflict are described as basically characteristic of human beings, what we actually have is a distortion which results from the methods of investigation used. What passes for a description of human nature is a description of individual or social pathology, or of human nature under artificial laboratory conditions which approximate pathology. Laboratory conditions frequently set up an artificial isolation that reproduces the segmentation of pathology.

> Freud . . . conceives of culture as a sublimation of repressed drives. This is a complete misapprehension of the creative trend of human nature.[a]

> The tendency to actualize itself is the . . . drive by which the organism is moved.
>
> The tendency to discharge any tension whatsoever is a characteristic expression of a defective organism of disease . . . the tendency to self-preservation is a characteristic of sick people and is a sign of . . . decay of life. For the sick person the only form of actualization of his capacities . . . is the maintenance of the existent state. This is not the tendency of the normal person.[b]

It is important in this connection to keep in mind Munroe's point that the same system of the organism may be described as need if the emphasis is on the inner state or as drive if the emphasis is on the external complement.[c] Neither of Munroe's descriptive terms, however, includes the wider meaning of goal carried by Goldstein's use of self-actualization and purpose.

In the discussion of the commonly accepted compensatory theory of personality, it was suggested that explanations of humor and laughter offer a peculiarly sensitive index to attitudes toward personality. Different interpretations of humor —including wit, laughter, the comic—focus the differences between the negative, tension-releasing, compensatory and the positive, tension-sustaining, purposive views of personality. Both agree on the sudden perception of discrepancy or incongruity as the essence of humor. They differ in the range of sources and meaning they discern in laughter and the comic.

The theory that the chief basis of laughter is enjoyment of the exposure and discomfiture of another person exhibits an impoverished view of personality.* According to the view of human nature as self-actualizing and goal-directed (in the wider sense), humor and laughter are part of the potential capacity of the human being for enjoyment—of himself, of and with other human beings, of and with the nonpersonal world. In a sick or truncated personality, or in a sick or truncated society, the sense of the ludicrous may become a substitute for weakness or aggression, and may be exercised at the expense of other people. But it need not be so limited. Humor can occur *with* other people, not as the enjoyment of power over, or at the expense of, other people. This is implied in the views of Schilder, Goldstein, and Schachtel, and is made more explicit by others who have given special attention to the varied sources and manifestations of humor.

> Laughter . . . in the child . . . is the sunny expression of satiety and enjoyment, of a spill-over of superfluous physical mental energy . . . laughter is rooted in the dispositions of play, gladness and sense of relief, and is by its nature happy and genial.
>
> The inadequacy of Bergson's explanation of laughter lies in . . . that he conceives only one kind of cause . . . for different types of laughter, one kind of incongruity or maladjustment as the spring of all laughter, viz., what is rigid, mechanical, or automatic encrusted on the living. . . .[a]

Boris Sidis, disparaged by Freudians, specifically takes issue with Freud's theory of laughter as based on scarcity of energy:

> . . . when some source of energy is tapped by an appropriate stimulus the result is joy and consequent laughter. In fact, we may say that the *release of reserve energy* is the source of all laughter.
>
> . . . wit is the opening of new horizons before the mental eye by means of the usual and the habitual associated with the unusual and unhabitual; and . . . by dissociation of elements and traits of

* See pp. 94-7.

the customary from their habitual surroundings and reassociation with the strange, the unusual, and uncustomary. . . . It is only when the customary . . . becomes transcended by a sudden manifestation and play of reserve energy . . . that true wit comes into being.* [a]

Murray is explicit in saying that the type of humor that consists in pleasure at the misfortune of those whom we envy is descriptive of only a certain type of laughter, not of all humor or of all laughter.[b] Humor that arises from enjoyment of the predicament of others may betoken a cynical self-interest that can be a warping experience for the observer as well as for the person observed.[c] This is not all of laughter. "When you laugh," says Turgenev, "you forgive and are ready to love." [d]

Regarding the nonpersonal world as a real world, not a shade world, includes being able to experience humor without personal mediation:†

The comic spirit is nourished and sustained by various kinds of incongruity; ideas and beliefs no less than persons and situations may be instances of the ludicrous. Ideas and belief, too, may be pretentious, pedantic, fantastic, bizarre, grotesque, inept, perverse, reckless, blind, and blatant.[e]

In relation to the nonpersonal world, as well as in relation to persons, it is possible to go beyond a compensatory theory of personality.

Amplification of Reward-Punishment Theories

Enlargement of a compensatory theory of personality development of necessity amplifies reward-punishment explanations of motivation. Stimulus-response mechanisms account accurately for certain specific and limited sorts of behavior, but fail to

* Boris Sidis, *The Psychology of Laughter,* used by permission of Appleton-Century-Croft, Inc., 1923, pp. 68-9, 70, 223.

† "Alone among the animals [man] is shaken with the beautiful madness called laughter; as if he had caught sight of some secret in the very shape of the universe hidden from the universe itself." (G. K. Chesterton, *The Everlasting Man,* Doubleday, Image Books, 1955, p. 35.)

explain (or even in some instances to recognize as important or accessible to understanding) experiences of the more pervasive sort, such as shame, under discussion here.

Theories of motivation built solely on reward and punishment are beginning to be widely questioned. Many psychologists regard hunger, so widely used as a motive in animal experiments, as an unfortunate model to explain human behavior.[a] Allport points out that, whatever may be true of a rat, we cannot predict the future behavior of a man unless we know his basic intentions, and that these basic intentions are by no means a stenciled copy of his previous expectancies and rewards.[b] Henry A. Murray insists that:

> More important than means-end learning . . . is goal-and goal-object learning; i.e., the process whereby an individual comes to some conclusions as to the relative values of different possible goals and goal objects. . . . Our knowledge of this latter process is very meagre, since science has taught Western intellectuals to keep out of the domain of values . . . and consequently, to leave the determination of social goals to chance and the operation of blind forces.[c]

No one has done more than Tolman to make use of animal models and animal experiments as means for understanding the behavior of human beings. It is, therefore, the more significant that his book, with the title *Purposive Behavior in Animals and in Men*,[d] points definitely beyond the pleasure principle. In it he concludes that the observed facts of learning call for a re-examination of stimulus-response laws for individuals of different degrees of intelligence, that both pre-Gestalt and Gestalt psychologists have tended to overlook the facts of individual differences, and that capacity laws must be added to stimulus laws of learning.[e] He states that purpose, by which he means more than goal in the narrow sense, is an objective fact which must be taken into account.

Harry F. Harlow makes an even stronger attack on the adequacy of theories of learning based on release of tension, reward and punishment. He believes that such "lax, ill-defined, subjective terms" as pain, pleasure, anxiety, and frustration should be dispensed with altogether; that strong tension or internal drive interferes with, instead of promoting, all but very limited aspects of learning, and that this is even truer of apes and of human beings than of animals lower in the phyletic scale, and truer of complex than of simpler forms of learning. In his view learning theories based on reduction of tension, reward and punishment neglect almost entirely the great diversity of the factors involved in learning in any one animal species and among different species. Desire to discover something in the outer world is of far greater importance for human beings than reduction of drive or release of tension.[a]

Alfred Adler's emphasis on the life-style of the individual beyond specific goals was the earliest psychoanalytic formulation to stress the purposive character of personality.[b] The importance of purpose as well as release of tension is now more generally recognized by analysts.

On the basis of anthropological evidence, Dorothy Lee specifically takes issue with theories of personality based on the hunger model and the view that action occurs only in answer to a need or a lack.

> . . . the Tikopio or the Kwoma infant, held and suckled without demand * in the mother's encircling arms . . . has no need for emotional response since his society is emotionally continuous with himself. . . . We create needs in the infant by withholding affection and then presenting it as a series of approvals for an inventory of achievements. . . . On the assumption that there is no emotional continuum, we withdraw ourselves, thus forcing the child to strive for emotional response and security.
>
> . . . for the Hopi . . . there is no external reward for being good, as this is taken for granted. It is evil which is external and intrusive.[c]

Goldstein finds that the reward-punishment theory of learning, like the compensatory theory of development, is inadequate because what it attributes to human nature is actually characteristic of sick or injured persons.

* There is a possibly ironical comment on our habits of thought in the fact that the more flexible feeding of infants practiced now as compared with thirty years ago is called "demand" feeding.

> [According to the stimulus-response theory] everything seems to be made for the preservation of the equilibrium state of the organism. But if the life of the organism consisted merely of an inter-play of elementary factors which kept each other in check, how could any movement, any dynamics, enter into the situation to give direction to behavior? And direction is what we actually find as the outstanding characteristic in the performances of an organism.[a]

> These [brain-damaged] patients must . . . follow the "pleasure principle." . . . [They] are only able to experience the pleasure of release of tension; they never appear to enjoy anything.[b]

One outcome of this emerging way of thinking is a profound alteration in the view of conflict in human life. For one school of thought conflict is something necessarily undesirable, to be got rid of. For the other it is part of the essence of life not to be done away with, even though it can become in certain areas excessive and impeding. Goldstein concludes that conflict or tension is not something to be deplored and resolved as soon as possible to restore a state of rest, but rather that the sustaining of tension is essential for any healthy living person.[c] It is the brain-injured,* the neurotically damaged person, who is unable to endure conflict, indecision, and the anxiety that may accompany conflict, who must always resolve indecision in some form of action.†

To a greater or lesser extent, anxiety accompanies conflict. Anxiety is, like shame, a pervasive experience deeply related to the core of the self. Anxiety has received much attention

* The terms brain-injured and brain-damaged refer to persons who have suffered physiological injury to the brain, not to those who show psychological disturbance with no manifest physiological injury.

† Goldstein's view of conflict as necessary for mental health is similar to that of D'Arcy Thompson on the necessity of stress in physical growth. "Partly associated with the . . . phenomenon [of functional adaptation] . . . is the very important physiological truth that a condition of *strain*, the result of a *stress*, is a direct stimulus to growth itself. This indeed is no less than one of the cardinal facts of theoretical biology. The soles of our boots wear thin, but the soles of our feet grow thick, the more we walk upon them." (D'Arcy Thompson, *On Growth and Form*, Macmillan, 1943, pp. 984-5.) Cf. Edmund Wilson's statement that the function of great art is not to resolve conflict but to express it in its full dimensions. (*The Triple Thinkers*, Oxford University Press, 1948.)

from psychoanalysts; every theory of anxiety distinguishes it from fear—roughly, fear being response to an actual threatening object in the external world, anxiety being less focused on any particular object, more related to the attitudes of the self. The distinction in German, referred to earlier, between *Ich fürchte etwas* and *Ich ängste mich* appears in some form in all theories of anxiety.

Freud's earlier explanations of anxiety emphasized physiological sources of anxiety, such as the flooding of the new system in the birth trauma of separation anxiety. He described repression as the source or cause of anxiety.[a] Later he came to regard anxiety not so much as the result of repression as the cause of repression, a signal of potential danger.[b]

Among non-Freudian psychoanalysts Sullivan has given most specific attention to the nature of anxiety; indeed, he regarded his study of anxiety as his major contribution to the understanding of personality development. Anxiety is, in Sullivan's view, a result of and a defense against insecurity. Insecurity is always associated with other persons, and is an outcome of deprivation in personal relations. Unlike fear, anxiety inhibits attention and alertness to the relevant factors in a situation. Arising from a lack in personal relations, it acts as a further disjunction. Thus anxiety which aims to prevent insecurity does so by actually increasing insecurity, more and more cutting off the individual from other persons as well as from the nonpersonal world.[c]

Goldstein agrees with Sullivan in viewing anxiety as a diffuse experience like shame, difficult to deal with, in part because it is nonlocalized either in the external world or in the self. Goldstein is explicit in saying that it is characteristic of the healthy person, and even more of the creative person, to be able to sustain conflict and doubt without an amount and kind of anxiety that is paralyzing. He agrees with Sullivan that, whereas fear may heighten the ability to act effectively, anxiety may paralyze the ability to act at all.[d] But he differs from Sullivan in his view that ability to live with some anxiety is necessary for the healthy person. The reason that the brain-damaged person has to act on the pleasure principle, must have immediate release of tension, and is unable to endure indecision or failure is that failure or postponement of decision confront him with an anxiety that is a threat to his very existence, the experience of being confronted with nothingness. A person who cannot live with indecision or anxiety has all his creative powers stunted because he is unable to deal with a range of what is possible, not actual.* Being able to live with what is possible is in one sense the test of being healthy or creative.

> Individuals differ as to how much anxiety they can bear. For a person with brain injury, the amount is very low, for a child it is greater, for the creative individual it is greatest.[a]

> [The] tendency toward actualization . . . can achieve its end only through a conflict with the opposing forces of the environment. This never happens without shock and anxiety. . . . The creative person, who ventures into many situations which expose him to shock, gets into these anxiety situations more often and more readily than the average person. . . . In the final analysis courage is . . . an affirmative answer to the shocks of existence, to the shocks which it is necessary to bear for the sake of realizing one's own nature. This form of overcoming anxiety requires the ability to view a single experience within a larger context, i.e., to assume the "attitude toward the possible," to maintain freedom of decision regarding different possibilities.[b]

In the search for the significant, emotion, capacity for thought, and ability to sustain tension and conflict combine to achieve human purposes. Thought is not a detour, a substitute, or a compensation, but an essentially human attribute. Consummation for the individual and working toward a more humane society both require the ability to sustain tensions in the immediate, to relate to other persons in more than obvious ways, and to act in terms of a range of the possible, of the evidence of things not seen.

* In the same way, Lewin stresses the danger of forcing a child too early to distinguish between reality and unreality; if he cannot entertain unrealities as possibilities his creative reach may be cramped. (Urie Bronfenbrenner, "Toward an Integrated Theory of Personality," in R. R. Blake and G. V. Ramsey, *Perception: An Approach to Personality*, Ronald Press, 1951, p. 213.)

Enlarged Possibilities in Human Relations

An interpretation of personality that includes purpose opens the way to understanding other people as persons, and to friendship, mutual discovery, and love in personal relations.

At least three views of other persons in relation to oneself have stood in the way of exploration of the meaning of mutual love.

One is Freud's conception of other human beings as objects that provide or withhold satisfaction of needs. Marx deplored the tendency of capitalist society to treat things as if they were living persons and persons as inanimate things. Freud's description of persons as objects that administer pleasure or pain tends to make a psychological necessity of what Marx accounted a defect of capitalism.[a] Freud's view that almost every intimate personal relation leaves a sediment of aversion and hostility* is closely allied, not only to Schopenhauer, whom he quotes, but to Proust, who believed that intimacy breeds contempt.

> It is the fate of sensual love to become extinguished when it is satisfied; for it to be able to last, it must . . . be mixed with purely tender components—with such, that is, as are inhibited in their aims.[b]

But even with tenderness, according to Freud, no one can tolerate too intimate an approach to another person.[c]

Fromm dissociates himself from Freud's view of other persons as objects or instruments of pleasure. But his use of "symbiotic" relations always in an invidious sense (turning the root meaning of symbiosis, living together in intimate association, into the derived meaning, parasitism) and his view that one must have a generalized love of everyone in order to love any one person can lead to a minimizing of the possibilities of mutual love between one person and another.†

* See pp. 90-1.

† Marcuse's criticism that Fromm's productive and nonproductive evaluations of personality simply embody the norms of our present performance society seems to me unjustified, particularly in view of Fromm's specific criticisms of capitalist institutions. (Marcuse, *Eros and Civilization*, pp. 250ff.)

A second conception that has interfered with the understanding of mutual love is the emphasis on hierarchies of superior and inferior status and functional roles that limit personal relations to some version of indulgent, deprivational, or indifferent.[a] Superior and inferior roles undoubtedly exist in most societies, including our contemporary market-place society, in which roles are vaguely defined but are perhaps more coercive because of their vagueness.* But hierarchies of roles are particular ways of phrasing human relations, not the only human relations possible. In a society dominated by power and anxiety, says Edith Weigert, "people meet each other in a variety of roles and 'take' each other by these roles: father and son, master and servant, husband and wife, seller and buyer, doctor and patient, teacher and pupil, one playmate and another. . . . These roles determine not only action, but already perception of a situation. . . . Success in a role means prestige, failure makes one lose face. Reputation, fame, or prestige are magic garments by which persons take hold of each other. . . . The roles [Jung's *persona,* mask] are disguises for the real Self."[b]

A third view that has blocked belief in the possibility of mutual discovery and love between persons was discussed in connection with the Freud-Benedict conception of shame. This is the stress on other persons as an audience who give or withhold approbation and ridicule. *Others* become a *They* who are apart from and over against the person involved. Certain possibilities in personal relations are already excluded, not only when the Others are regarded as a ridiculing and unfriendly audience, but when they are regarded as any kind of an *audience.*†

It is possible for other persons to become more than objects to release tensions or to satisfy needs, or embodiments of particular role or status relations, or than an audience over against oneself. They can be persons, ends in themselves, and only if they are so conceived are certain kinds of human relations pos-

* See pp. 18, 19.

† George Herbert Mead appears to regard others in the role of audience as essential to the development of a sense of oneself. (*Mind, Self & Society,* University of Chicago Press, 1934.)

sible. If we take seriously the possibility of relating to other persons as persons, then seeing them primarily as need-satisfying objects, or in terms of their particular status or role relations to oneself, or as approving or disapproving audience is as limited as seeing personality primarily in terms of release of tension, return to quiescence, and self-preservation.

Schilder rejects the idea of hierarchy as either basic or necessary in human relations, and conceives mutuality as a genuine possibility for human beings who are as essentially social in desiring other human beings as they are individual. A full love relation comprises the appreciation of another person's personal and sexual qualities. Relating to another person in terms of superiority and inferiority, aggression and submission can only interfere with mutual discovery and love.[a] Schilder's statement that other persons should be treated as persons seems the ultimate platitude, but it is a platitude almost as much neglected by clinical psychologists and psychoanalysts as by social institutions. For some psychoanalysts the person is the patient in his office; other persons in the environment of the patient—family, friends, professional associates—are so many objects who foster or interfere with the patient's well-being. But there is some denial of human dignity with the loss of a perspective in which each person matters. In Schilder's view

> If one tries to consider other human beings from the point of view of how much gratification they can give to one's wish of being passively loved and admired, the other people do not remain personalities but are merely schemes. In addition to that, they become more or less threats . . . full human relations are not possible unless we respect the independent existence of other human beings.[b]

To see sexual desire in terms of release of tension and loved persons as objects to satisfy need is, Schachtel believes, a sign of neuroticism. Such relations to persons do indeed breed satiety and leave a residue of dislike. But love can be potentially inexhaustible and lasting, instead of subsiding with the satisfaction of the need. Such love finds its fulfillment "not in a discharge of tension but, rather, in a maintenance of it, in sustained and ever renewed acts of relating to the beloved person." [a]

Rorschach rejected the inevitability of a hierarchical view of the human enterprise, and hoped that like the fact that introversion was for so long regarded as pathological, insistence on the necessity of hierarchy could be recognized as a particular cultural, historical phenomenon, a characteristic of what he called the materialistic extratensive epoch.[b] Just as he rejected the necessity for using categories that are some version of the ladder of success, so he refused to subsume human capacity for joy under either compensation for inadequacy or triumph over others. He, too, stressed the possibility of renewed mutual discovery between persons as an enlargement, not a contradiction, of individual freedom; and of capacity for joy in and with others as a basic attribute of human beings. Unlike Bertram Lewin, who treats elation as only pathological,[c] Rorschach regarded it as a mood that, in contrast to depression, which is constricting, releases and expands capacity for fresh experience and insight.[d]

Harry Stack Sullivan built his whole theory of personality development on the nature of an individual's relations with other persons. He recognized the possibility of viewing individual freedom and membership in a social group as essential to each other rather than as antithetical. He believed, not only that the character of the individual self is shaped by its particular personal relations, but that apart from personal relations there is no self; the continuing being of a person is continuously interpersonal. He concluded that an individual can be understood only in terms of the whole system of social relations that has produced him; the doctor cannot diagnose individual ills without taking the whole environment of the patient's relations with others into account; the total interpersonal situation of a patient in hospital, in neighborhood, or in the wider society is more important in effecting a cure than any particular doctor or therapy. Mutuality, in Sullivan's view, is so essential for good personal relations that it should extend even to the relation between analyst and patient. Indeed, this equality of exchange and mutual discovery was for him the most important element in therapy. In dealing with students, with patients, or with persons in any group, the first step, he believed, is to see the world through their eyes, to enter into what they are trying to do, however strange their behavior may appear. Genuine communication is impossible on any other basis.[a]

A similar emphasis on treating patients first of all as human beings to be respected appears in the work of Frieda Fromm-Reichmann[b] and of Marguerite Sechehaye.[c] Both open up extraordinary possibilities in showing what can be accomplished by entering imaginatively into the lives of other persons whose illness has cut them off from human relations and by finding ways of establishing communication with them.

The central importance that Schilder, Sullivan, and others ascribe to the quality of the relations between persons, and to the possibility of mutual respect, discovery, and love between them, derives from their observations of individuals. There is some evidence, based upon study of social groups, to suggest that the conception of a society built less upon role-playing and the giving and withholding of favor, a society that makes it more possible for mutuality to develop between persons, is not an impossible ideal.

It would appear that there are societies where the self is less separate from others than in our own, where individualism does not rest upon a polarizing of the individual and of society, where the enabling rather than the limiting aspects of the social group and of the culture are more recognized and stressed. Handlin describes the "old world" of the peasants as one in which there was a relationship of solidarity among all natural things. This feeling of solidarity and support prevailed among human beings in a particular area and extended to all living things. "If the birds flew away to the woods, then the snow would soon decide to fall. . . . All the objects of nature were engaged in growth." [d] Helen Mims has explored the sense of individual realization through the bonds of the community in medieval communities, particularly in England and Spain. These communities confronting the expanding state included peasant and village communities, walled cities, unwalled communities of cities and land, parishes, and guilds. They were often referred to as neighborhoods; back of each neighborhood lay a wholeness of living together. It was the strength, depth, and range of the attachments that tied the individual to a particular community as distinguished from all others.[a]

Dorothy Lee has described this mutually enhancing relation between individual and social group in Greece, ancient and modern:

> Individualism is prized and rampant; yet there is no atomization. Self-esteem is paramount, and rests on freedom and self-dependence; yet Greeks do not seek freedom from the family. . . . Foremost in the Greek's view of the self is his self-esteem . . . the Greek *philotimo.* . . . Everyone has his *philotimo,* as an individual, as a member of a family, and most of all as a Greek. On this rests Greek individualism, since it is sheer being which is respected, not position in the world or achievement . . . relationships of interdependence, of leader and followers . . . are not cast in the mould of superiority and inferiority. Inferiority comes only with the forfeiting of the *philotimo.*[b]

It is necessary to the Greek to be able to feel shame in order to have self-esteem.[c]

Dodds, when he says that "the liberation of the individual from the bonds of clan and family is one of the major achievements of Greek rationalism," [d] seems to use bonds only in the sense of restraint and to show only a limited understanding of a culture where structured interpersonal relations are essential to the freedom and self-realization of the individual. This is something different from the *subordination* of the individual to the group.

It may be that it is only in societies, like our Western post-Renaissance society, that regard individual freedom as atomism that guilt, a separate, individual act that transgresses a barrier, attracts more attention than shame, a falling short of ideals, and that it is only in such a society that the social group is looked upon as a threat to individual freedom.[e] We must remember that it is a special version of life which regards society as external to the individual, mother love as something "given" to the child, emotional "needs" as something that must be felt and "met," the social group as a series of links rather than a continuum. There may be wide differences in the range of what is conceived as possible according to whether one starts with the assumption of separate individuals and then considers how they may be linked together or starts with the assumption of related persons and then considers how they may develop individuality within the group.

The possibility of personal self-realization in and through relations with others and of a society in which alienation is overcome suggests Rousseau's, Hegel's, and Marx's vision of the good life in which self-realization and relations with other persons in one's social group will be not antithetical but mutually enhancing.

There is a paradox and a problem involved for anyone who believes that individual self-realization and group welfare can come increasingly to enhance each other. But it is not essentially, as is sometimes alleged, a *Marxian* problem. It is a problem, also, for Erikson, for Fromm, for Marcuse, for anyone who believes in the possibilities of democracy, anyone who believes that the integrity and freedom of the self and of the social group may be, not Platonic opposites or distributions of an economic scarcity of well-being, but enlargements of each other. The possibility under discussion here is one of a society in which diversities in ranges of inner life and of personal relations will find expression and social support. The whole animus and direction of such a society would be different from the kind of group organization described, for example, by William H. Whyte, Jr., or in certain religious groups in which individual diversity is submerged in the group.[a]

The ability to enter into relations of intimacy and mutuality opens the way to experiences in which the self expands beyond its own limitations in depth of feeling, understanding, and insight.[b] One's own identity may be, not weakened, but strengthened by the meaning one has for others in one's group and by respect for these other persons as distinct individuals.

This experience involves the risks of trusting oneself to other persons instead of regarding them in object, status, role, or audience relations. It also means not allowing disappointment in response from another person to lead to a denial of the expectation and possibility of love.

> . . . it takes a certain audacity on the part of the philosopher-psychologist to talk about Love. . . . Love is so much pushed into the background that many people do not believe in the . . . existence of Love, or consider it to be only a comforting illusion of poetry. . . . There is a deeply ingrained embarrassment or shame even in admitting a sincere yearning for Love. In our present-day culture there is no great difficulty in talking about sexuality, particularly if it is considered as a successful performance. . . . But Love is deeply taboo.
>
> In the transcendence of Love there is no anxiety nor struggle for self-assertion, for in the we-ness the Self is received as a gift of grace.[a]

A person who is unable to love cannot reveal himself.

View of the Outer World

All that has gone before implies that the development of individual identity must be understood, not in a "shadow-world," but in a world conceived in its full dimensions—personal and nonpersonal.

It has become at least a verbal commonplace that the real world within which the individual must be understood must be the human world of his milieu, his social situation, his culture. If we begin with studying individuals we now find ourselves studying society; if we begin with society we cannot avoid studying the individuals who compose it. There are institutes and conferences on human behavior and social relations to promote *rapprochement* among psychoanalysis and psychology and the various social sciences, especially anthropology and sociology. The term psychosocial units has come into use. Even Geza Roheim, who has been most emphatic among psychoanalysts in condemning the cultural approach, has incorporated some of its concepts in his later writing.[b]

There is still some tendency, however—for those who would

consider no care too great to lavish on the relation between the libido and the various defenses of the ego, or on the development of the different self-dynamisms, or on learning theories—to act as if once they have decided to recognize the social situation as essential for understanding of personality, *its* dynamisms can be understood with relative ease. Psychoanalysts and psychologists are not always aware that the same sense of humility and of the complexity of the data that they would regard as essential in interpreting a dream are required also for any understanding of economic, political, and historical structures and trends. (It should be noted that this same attitude in reverse is shown by many social scientists: a political scientist aware of the complexities in his own field may think that "the psychological factors" can be added as a fairly simple postscript to the study of institutions, or even that "psychologizing" is an irrelevant diversion.) Heinz Hartmann, as a psychoanalyst, says that "in contrast to some other schools of psychology, psychoanalysis includes within its scope of interest the structure of reality. . . . We must accept social reality as a factor in its own right." [a] But it remains true that many psychoanalysts, as well as many psychologists, work as if, having decided to include within their scope of interest "the structure of reality," the task is essentially done; and that the majority of psychoanalysts and psychologists who stress adaptation as a desirable end regard the reality that we must accept or adjust to as the reality of bourgeois society in this particular historical epoch.

There are some, nevertheless, who without mastering the complexities of the various social sciences at least recognize that the complexities exist with their own requirements for detailed knowledge and understanding, and that the social situation cannot simply be added on as an appendage to the study of the individual. Awareness of these complexities does not mean that every investigator must be omnicompetent or omniscient; there can be awareness of and respect for the problems of another area of specialization without intimate knowledge.

Schilder never loses sight of the fact that the world in which human beings live and move and think is a real world, not a shade world.

> Psychoanalysis has repeatedly tried to explain objects and the recognition of them as a projection of one's own tendencies. That means putting the cart before the horse. There is a world and there are love objects which impress the individual and give rise to certain tendencies in him. . . . We need an outer world, we want to have power over this outer world, we want to re-create this world into its true self.[a]

Adler and Karen Horney, in general terms, and Fromm and Erikson, more specifically, have stressed the fact that understanding of the meaning of human behavior and of the development of individual personality must be related to knowledge of the specific social milieu that has shaped it. Erikson is emphatic in saying that knowledge of cultural conditions shaping personality needs to go beyond the common-sense acknowledgment that such writers as Hartmann, Kris, and Loewenstein[b] "find sufficient." [c] Abram Kardiner has attempted to relate special kinds of character development with specific social demands.[d]

Less generally recognized than the importance of the social world of people for understanding the individual is the importance of the nonpersonal world. The real world is a world of things as well as a world of persons. This again seems like the most obvious platitude. But it is widely affirmed by Neo-Freudian psychologists that interest in or relations to inanimate objects can be formed only through or after relations to human objects. Art and science are sublimations of thwarted drives in relation to other human beings; the discrepancies that give rise to humor and laughter are always personal or always have personal relevance. In the valuable insistence by psychologists in recent years on the crucial role of relations to mother, family, and social group in the development of the individual, the relation of the individual to the real, nonpersonal world has sometimes tended to be overlooked.

Paradoxically, it is Sullivan, with his explicit insistence on the central importance of personal relations, who has been a leader in directing attention to the inescapable importance of the nonpersonal world for the development of the individual.

In our heightened awareness of the human relevance of every experience we tend to lose sight of the fact that there are experiences, natural objects, works of art that have significance apart from their human associations and import. Hamlet's concern with the players springs not only from his intent to use them to reveal the true nature of Claudius, but from his interest in acting as acting, and theater as theater. Proust's, and in a different way Gide's, achievement consists in turning experiences almost unbearably poignant in their human import into works of art that have form and interest of their own. In Gerard Manley Hopkins the world of nature, of music, of sound and the cadence of words aroused a passion more often called forth only by other human beings, and of an intensity rarely found even in human relations.

Schachtel's studies of "The Dynamic Perception of Form" [a] and "The Development of Focal Attention" [b] beautifully unfold the process of growing awareness of the world of nonpersonal reality. Perception is at every moment colored by the emotional and intellectual life-style of the perceiver and by what his particular social situation and historical period have taught him to see. But it occurs most fully when insistent personal concerns can be held in suspension enough to allow concentration on the thing observed.

By focal attention, as distinguished from other forms of attention, I designate man's capacity to *center* his attention on an object fully, so that he can perceive or understand it from *many sides*. . . . Focal attention is the main instrument which . . . enables man to progress from the primitive mental activity of wishing or wanting . . . to a grasp of reality.
' . . . focal attention plays a most important role in the gradual emergence and constitution of the object world (reality) and of the sense of self.[c]

Originally, object was that which is *ob-jectum*—that is, the thing thrown before the mind, the thing which one encounters. . . . In this paper, the word object is used only for the object that exists independent of man's needs. . . . It has an existence of its own.

In contrast to Freud's view, I believe that thought has two ancestors rather than one—namely, motivating needs *and* a distinctively human capacity, the relatively autonomous capacity for object interest. Focal attention is the tool, the distinctively human equipment, by means of which the capacity for object interest can be realized.[a]

The work of Rudolf Arnheim similarly takes in its full dimensions the importance of the real world, personal and nonpersonal. Arnheim stresses less than Schachtel the extent to which the individual life-style of a person determines what he perceives, and more the degree to which there are correspondences between any perceiving person and the world of persons and things perceived. On the basis of the evidence of Gestalt psychology he concludes that there are certain forms in the external world that appear no matter how great the variation in individual and cultural factors which affect perception.[b]

Another aspect of the real world that is beginning to receive more attention from psychologists and social scientists is historical change. Neglect of history has arisen in part, as noted above, from too narrow a conception of what constitutes historical understanding—from the invalid contrasts between history as an art as opposed to a science and between history as dealing with individual events in contrast to science, which deals with laws. The metaphor "laws" itself, as Frederick J. Teggart has said, has been an unfortunate one as it has led us to make the wrong kinds of demands in searching for the meaning of historical data.[c]

What is often referred to as a contradiction in Marxian theory, namely, that there are certain necessities in historical development but that men are, nevertheless, exhorted to make their own history, is a problem and a paradox, but (like the complementariness of individual self-realization and group welfare) it is not an essentially *Marxian* paradox. It is a problem for anyone who believes that there are discoverable and, at least to some extent, predictable sequences in human history, but who believes that the purposes and actions of men are part of history and that they can, to however slight a degree, alter the course of events. "The historian's business is to reveal the less obvious features hidden from a careless eye in the present situation. What history can bring to moral and political life is a trained eye for the situation in which one has to act." [a]

From different sides there comes evidence that social scientists and some psychologists are beginning to overcome their distrust of any attempt to trace historical sequences and to realize the necessity of historical dimensions for the understanding of present situations. More humbly and slowly than a century ago, historians are renewing the search for hypotheses that may throw light on relations among events and social developments. In 1954 the Social Science Research Council published a detailed analysis of the kinds of problems presented by the study of history and the kinds of enlargement of possibilities for the other social sciences that use of historical method can provide.[b] Margaret Mead in defining the requirements that are essential for responsible research on "national character" in *Anthropology Today* includes among them "recourse to a known sequence of historical events." [c] Even ten years ago it would have been possible to assemble the kinds of materials which appear in this volume with an almost exclusive emphasis on "synchronic" studies at the expense of historical or "dyachronic" studies. Paul Lazarsfeld's suggestion that a commission be formed consisting of historians and public-opinion experts to advise on what issues are relevant for opinion-poll studies[d] reveals a recognition that predictive opinion polls may have value for future historians, and even, perhaps, that some historical perspective might have value for opinion pollsters.

Even with the quickening recognition of the necessity for historical understanding, however, Erikson is still exceptional among his fellow students in psychoanalysis and comparative culture in his emphasis on the necessity for including study of the processes of history and of the concreteness of a present historical situation in the study of personality and culture. In 1946, writing on "Ego Development and Historical Change," he said that it is necessary to know both the particular historical situation in which the child's ego developed and the changing historical reality that has influenced psychoanalytic concepts and theory.[e] In 1952 he again urged psychologists to be aware that psychologies and psychologists are a product of their historical situation as much as historians are subject to the laws of psychology.[a] Erikson believes that psychologists should be aware of the historical as well as the psychological roots of the human characteristics they study. The current concept of the rejecting mother, for example, which has become a psychiatric cliché, Erikson thinks cannot be understood in psychological terms alone but must be seen as a part of the development of the conditions of American pioneer life and the particular character of the American Puritan tradition.[b]

Revival of Psychological Interest in the Self

Particularly pertinent to experiences of shame, as *self*-consciousness which can become a revelation of identity, is the increasing appearance in psychological and psychoanalytic writing of some version of the self. There was a period, now apparently coming to an end, when the self was discussed more by philosophers and sociologists[c] than by psychologists. Consideration of the questions Who am I? Where do I belong? tended to be banned from psychology as unscientific and not lending themselves to operationalism and experiment.[d] At present these questions have re-entered psychological discussion and are granted at least reluctant recognition.

The self goes by many names, and the word self has many meanings. Almost every psychologist has certain terms referring to the self which he defines elaborately, others which he slips in as if everyone knew what they meant. What for one is obvious, for another needs exhaustive explanation. And the categories of explanation or lack of explanation in which the same term appears are in many cases contradicted or reversed by different writers.

Hume referred to the self only to deny its existence. This is true also of some contemporary positivists and pragmatists. Almost every psychologist uses the word individual without definition, even if he considers it necessary to explain the word organism elaborately.

Some psychologists give careful definitions of personality.[a] For them, as for most psychologists, personality is the most inclusive term to indicate all aspects of an individual from biological through social, a more inclusive term than self, ego, or character.* Personality is a term somewhat less used by psychoanalytically oriented writers. Their usual terms are personality structure, as applied to an individual, character structure, as applied to a society, although even these terms are sometimes reversed in meaning.[b]

Self and ego are still more slippery in usage. The terms self and ego slide around like the shiny balls under glass in a child's puzzle, which no matter how the board is tilted refuse to stay lodged in any particular hollows. Self is sometimes used, as William James used it,[c] as the more inclusive concept of which the ego is a part, by some writers as almost synonymous with personality.[d] Other psychologists refer to the self as a part of the personality, a subsystem or a schema, an object of experience or consciousness, not a conscious agent or knower, with the ego as somewhat loosely, a part of the self.[e] Some reverse this usage and describe the self as less comprehensive than the ego; as an active, conscious agent, the phenomenal representation of the ego, a core that with the addition of attitudes, ideals, motives, and values becomes the ego and that with still other additions becomes the personality.[f]

Freud makes almost no use of the term self. Sullivan uses the term self-dynamism to emphasize the complex and never-completed process of development. Jung contrasts the *animus* and *anima,* the male and female components, that are the sources of the self, with the *persona,* the mask with which the root self covers itself and which it presents to the world. He reserves the term self for the integration of all aspects of the personality, conscious and unconscious. The self in Jung's usage is a lifetime achievement, neither a psychological given nor one aspect of a more comprehensive personality. The more organ-

* In contemporary usage personality can stand for both the external, superficial characteristics of the individual, or for his intrinsic, inner nature, or—as is perhaps most frequent—for both combined.

ized and outwardly directed *persona* is only a part of it. For Horney and Fromm there is a real or true or spontaneous self that is contrasted both with an extravagant self-image or idealized self and with the conventional self which attempts to conform to the world.

In distinguishing self from ego, many psychologists refer to "the Freudian use of 'ego.'" But Freud himself used ego both in a wide sense as roughly synonymous with the person and in a narrower sense as one psychological system, distinguished from the id and the superego. In this second usage, whereas Asch uses self as a part of a more inclusive ego, Freud uses ego (including in his later writings unconscious factors) as part of a more inclusive, although unnamed, self. Federn, who gives the most elaborate Freudian explanations of the ego, defines it as "the lasting or recurring psychical continuity of the body *and* mind in respect of space, time, and causality." [a] Bronfenbrenner believes that the phenomena referred to by Freud as ego (in the wider sense) and by Lewin as self are comparable, if not identical.[b]

This suggestion of a few of the many diverse meanings that have become attached to the words self and ego is not intended to underline the complexity of the present semantic difficulties in regard to these terms. Rather, it indicates that many different schools of thought are tending to recognize and converge upon the question of sense of identity under discussion here.* The contemporary interest of Freudians in ego psychology, Jung's distinction of the *animus* and *anima* from the masking *persona,* Adler's stress on the importance of individual life style, Horney's real self, and Fromm's true self—each is in its different way a recognition of the present importance of the search for identity. The psychoanalytic emphasis on psychological systems related to internal stimuli is beginning to be combined with the emphasis of academic psychology on systems related to external stimuli in an effort to understand how these systems function together in an individual to form a sense of himself.

* Cf. pp. 204-07 for discussion of Erikson's use of the term identity, which combines some of the meanings other investigators have given to self and ego.

Thus far nothing has been said about the part played by the ideal one has for oneself in developing a sense of one's own identity. But it is readily apparent that the ideal of who one might or desires to be or become has important bearing on one's feeling about who one is.

The confusion of terms and of meanings surrounding the uses of superego, self-image, self-ideal, ego-ideal, ideal self is perhaps even greater than that which confounds the uses of self and ego. It extends to lack of any agreement as to whether projecting an ideal self-image is desirable or undesirable. It leads to assumptions, often unstated, as to whether the ideal self-image can be entirely traced to identifications with the parents or with the parents' ideal, or to the combining of the various roles prescribed by one's culture.

However confused in its various uses, the question of the meaning and role of the ideal self-image is at the core of Piers' distinction between guilt and shame—that guilt is the transgression of a prescribed boundary or taboo, shame a falling short of one's own ideal, which may or may not occur in the presence of others.* The role of the self-ideal goes to the heart of the search for identity.

For Ortega y Gasset the self-ideal is something that transcends actual life experience. He goes beyond any psychologist's conception of the ideal self in asserting that the "I" to be realized is something other and more than "body, soul, consciousness, or character." The "I" is "a vital design," a "single programmatic personage who must be realized." "Life is essentially a desperate struggle to succeed in being in fact that which we are in design. . . . To live is to be outside oneself, to realize oneself. The vital program, which each of us irremediably is, overpowers environment to lodge itself there." [a]

Freud made little use of the concept of self- or ego-ideal after he developed his view of the superego as one of the three subsystems of the personality. He had made reference to an ego-ideal in "On Narcissism" (1914).[b] Here it was a derivative of early narcissism. The superego was developed later in Freud's

* See p. 22.

thought as a derivative of identification with the parents or with the parents' ideals.[a] The superego with its emphasis on the negative, forbidding, censoring aspects of conscience was more prominent in Freud's thought.[b]

For Jung the self-ideal possibly tends to slip away somewhere between the *animus* and the *anima* (which together as the "shadow" comprise the unconscious aspects of the self) and the more conscious, adaptive, social-role aspects of the self, which he calls the *persona*.[c] Munroe identifies Jung's adaptively organized image of the self, the *persona*, with the self-image.[d]

In Horney's terms the self-ideal or idealized image of the self is contrasted unfavorably with the real self; the idealized image of the self tends to be neurotic, an ideal that interferes with the pursuit of authentic, attainable, realistic goals.[e] Sullivan's system makes way for, although he does not explicitly discuss, the conflict among various self-images. Both satisfaction of bodily needs and security in relation to other persons enter into his conception of the development of the self-images and of the self-system. Emphasis on the pluralism of the various dynamic systems that compose the personality runs through his entire theory.

Others tend to confine the self-image as well as the self to an internalization of roles, or system of role expectations.[f] Too great fluency in the use of the terms role and status marks many discussions of the relations of social roles to the image of the ideal self. Finding oneself is something different from finding one's role or roles, and if this distinction is lost, we have blocked off an essential road to the understanding of identity.*

The Freudian concepts of introjection (internalization) and identification bring us closer to the question of how the ideal self-image is formed. Former love objects are introjected by the self, conceptualized as identifications, lose their independence, and become integrated, on the one hand as the ego, on the other as an ideal or superego.[g]

These questions remain: How are identifications with parental ideals and prescribed social roles selected, combined, and extended in ways that enable an individual to say: This is I?

* Cf. pp. 184-95.

And are there identifications beyond those of his immediate culture that help to frame his ideas of what he is and what he wants to be? These questions will be discussed further in the next chapter.

New Ways in Language

Language, and the variety of ways in which it can be used, has special importance for the realization of identity. The child as he learns to speak acquires a further delineation of himself—a taking on of responsibility for what he says, a further means of entering into relations with other persons, and a sharpening of perception of certain aspects of the world.*

I have spoken of the difficulty of finding a language that can communicate such experiences as shame and a sense of identity, and of the fact that the present prevailing emphasis on perfecting a language of signs (indispensable as such a language is and will continue to be for some purpose), may retard exploration of other possibilities in language. Insistence on unambiguous, minute precision of language as the sole criterion of responsible use not only diverts attention from, but precludes by axiom, the development of a language through which more multifarious, complex, experiences can be expressed.

Although the attempt to develop a language of fixed, unequivocal signs is currently in the ascendant, not only among psychologists, social scientists, and exponents of symbolic logic (by whom symbol is used in a limited meaning that approaches that of signal or sign), but also in contemporary linguistics, there are, nevertheless, some indications of recognition of the more varied, symbolic possibilities of language. Development of such possibilities should supplement, never replace, the uses of language as sign and as a more limited sort of symbol.

From a variety of sources comes a realization that the importance of certain experiences cannot be measured by the exact-

* As Schachtel has pointed out (see pp. 247-8), acquiring of language frequently means a dulling and conventionalizing of perception. But it is possible for use of words to quicken, not to deaden, awareness.

ness with which they can be codified and communicated through an unequivocal language of signs, and a consequent endeavor to find ways through the barrier of reliance on sign language and across the gulf of lack of other language.

Some of the interest in exploring the symbolic possibilities of language arises from an awareness of the extent to which not only what can be communicated but also what is perceived is affected by the forms of languages and the meanings carried by them. Edward Sapir in 1929 stated what has come to be known as the Sapir-Whorf hypothesis: that language functions, not simply as a device for reporting and communicating experience, but also as a way of defining experience in different cultures.[a]

> . . . the "real world" is to a large extent unconsciously built up on the language habits of the group. No two languages are ever sufficiently similar to be considered as representing the same social reality. The worlds in which different societies live are distinct worlds, not merely the same world with different labels attached.[b]

> Language is at one and the same time helping and retarding us in our exploration of experience, and the details of these processes of help and hindrance are deposited in the subtler meanings of different cultures.[c]

This stress on language as affecting, and to some extent determining, what is perceived and how experience is interpreted includes the analogies implied by the language as well as what is directly said. Something different is implied, for example, by saying "The grass is waved by the wind" or "The wind causes the grass to wave" than by "The grass waves in the wind." [d]

Benjamin Whorf and Harry Hoijer have carried Sapir's studies further by their work on the varieties of meanings explicit and implicit in language. "Every culture," says Whorf, "is a vast pattern system . . . in which is culturally ordained the forms and categories by which the personality not only communicates, but analyzes nature, notices or neglects types of relationship and phenomena, channels his reasoning, and builds the house of his consciousness. . . . Science, poetry, love are alike in being 'flights' above and away from the . . . world of literal reference. . . . Western culture has gone . . . farthest in determined thoroughness of provisional analysis, and farthest in determination to regard it as final." [a]

It is commonly asserted that if other cultures which we designate as more primitive have developed language forms and meanings that may seem to extend the range of experience in some directions, Western civilization owes to Aristotelian categories and their derivatives the development of Western science, and that this means that whatever the charm some of these other world views may have, we can learn little from them.* Whorf's view is that some of these other languages actually express scientific concepts that we assume can be expressed only in our Western forms, and also that some of their ways of expression can extend the range of our own science. He states that careful study of the Hopi language has convinced him that it contains no words or grammatical structures that refer to time, or to past, present, and future in the sense we assume to be universal, but that, nevertheless, it is capable of accounting for, in a pragmatic or operational sense, all observable phenomena of the universe.

> . . . if MYSTICAL be . . . a term of abuse in the eyes of a modern Western scientist, it must be emphasized that these underlying abstractions . . . of the Hopian metaphysics are, from a detached viewpoint, equally . . . justified pragmatically and experimentally, as compared to the flowing time and static space of our own metaphysics, which are *au fond* equally mystical.[b]

The Hopi conceive time and motion in the objective realm in a purely operational sense . . . so that the element of time is not separated from whatever element of space enters into the operations.

* Compare with this view Whatmough's statement that "It can easily be shown, on purely linguistic evidence, that those linguistic features which underlie our modern Western civilization—concepts such as mass, force, energy, volume, time and space, gravity and so forth—have evolved from older stages of Indo-European languages which were not at all unlike those of many American Indian dialects . . . in which modern scientific expressions could not have been formed. Aristotelian Greek could no more have formulated modern chemistry or physics than Arabic or Hopi; nor can modern English cope with some of the theory in articulate discourse, but only in formulae." (Joshua Whatmough, *Language: A Modern Synthesis,* St. Martin's Press, 1956, p. 186.)

. . . 'Events' in [a] distant village can be compared to any events in one's own village only by an interval of magnitude that has both time and space forms in it. . . . Hopi, with its preference for verbs, as contrasted to our own liking for nouns, perpetually turns our propositions about things into propositions about events.[a]

Dorothy Lee reports a somewhat similar ordering of time and space, whole and parts, among the Trobrianders.[b] In the society of the Wintu she finds that the whole, rather than the part, is taken as the given.

For the Wintu . . . essence, or quality, is generic and found in nature; it is permanent and remains unaffected by man. Form is imposed by man through act of will.

The particular . . . exists, not in nature, but in the consciousness of the speaker. What to us is a class, a plurality of particulars, is to him a mass or a quality or an attribute.[c]

. . . the Wintu conceive of the self not as strictly limited or defined, but as a concentration, at most, which gradually fades and gives place to the other. Most of what we call other for us, is for the Wintu completely or partially or upon occasion, identified with the self.[d]

Anselm Strauss analyzes the importance in our own society of shifts in language patterns in ordering our perception of the world and of ourselves. The way one behaves, how one feels, and what one does in relation to particular other persons, objects, and institutions frequently depend upon what is singled out by giving it a name and by the connotations of the particular names used. This applies especially to status and role relations, but to other relations as well. The renaming of a particular social phenomenon may bring about a change in behavior toward it. The way time is conceived and divided in a society, the way processes of development and attainment are phrased, what is designated as normal and abnormal behavior—all are outcomes of ways of behaving, and in turn reinforce these forms of behavior.[e]

The view that perception and conceptualization of reality are so largely determined by the structure and meaning of language—and the Sapir-Whorf hypothesis in particular—has been criticized as underestimating universal human factors in ways of ordering reality and overestimating the differences in what is expressed by different languages. Lewis Feuer says flatly that a language may be at most "a minor agency of syntactical resistance or syntactical propensity toward certain philosophic views. It has none of the properties of importance with which it is endowed by linguistic philosophers." [a] He maintains that the same philosophies have arisen among peoples with radically different languages, that the most diverse types of philosophy have arisen among people who use the same language, and that the extent to which one language is untranslatable into another has been greatly exaggerated.[b] But he recognizes that, although the syntax of any language is composed both of forms and distinctions that correspond to natural realities and those that are projected by the language upon realities, different languages do emphasize different relations of men to nature and make some aspects of reality more readily accessible and more important in organizing social life than others.[c]

This last is really the central point of the Sapir-Whorf hypothesis and, although it may at times have been overstated, Feuer's analysis neither denies nor refutes it. It is not necessary to ignore the existence of characteristics common to all human beings and expressed in their various languages in order to recognize the wide range of forms of these linguistic expressions. These varying expressions select for emphasis different aspects of life. Any language in use is to some degree *adequate* for expression of human wants and of interpretation of the world, and there can still be wide differences in degrees and kinds of adequacy and in the ranges of experiences that can find expression beyond minimal adequacy.

On the basis of a much more complex analysis than Feuer's, Whatmough takes issue with the Sapir-Whorf hypothesis, or at least with the more extreme claims made for it. He believes that: life fashions language; the assertion that grammatical categories impose compulsion upon action is not justified historically since language has often pointed a way out from restriction on action; the argument of a fundamentally different time concept in Hopi and Indo-European languages does not hold; language if unfettered by a dead tradition "solves its own problems"; diversity of languages does not mean a diversity of the aspects in which the world is seen.[a] Whatmough is more interested in the development of languages in themselves, and in comparing and contrasting them, than in their relation to psychology and to society; his statements may underestimate the selective effects of language on aspects of reality perceived as much as some of Sapir's may overestimate it. He may actually underplay the power of language.

The relevance of these questions on the nature of language for understanding such experiences as shame and the sense of identity is that the trend toward emphasis on a language of fixed signs (which has been essential for, and has been in turn strengthened by, the development of natural science) has led to disparagement of a language which can express awareness of other ranges of experience. Graham Hough commented on the efforts of the logical positivists to assimilate language to mathematics and the records of empirical science and the condemnation of all other uses of language as "nonsense":

> . . . if this view is correct, the analysis of nonsense assumes a hitherto unsuspected importance. For though many of the propositions [classified] . . . as nonsense have indeed no bearing on anything, many of them have a powerful effect on the way people actually behave. Nobody goes to prison because he believes the snark is a boojum, but some people have done so because they believe that killing is wrong. If these statements are both nonsense, at least they are nonsense of very different kinds.[b]

Iredell Jenkins believes that the insistence of the logical positivists that many of the propositions most significant to men are really meaningless has resulted in substituting a denial of important problems for investigation of them, and has impoverished not only the uses of language but the concept of man. Other modes of behavior than scientific inquiry (such as emotional, moral, aesthetic, religious)* are treated as trivial or

* J. Varendonck, in speaking of the fact that daydreams do not lend themselves readily to communication, says that the concentration in Western culture on rational consciousness has blunted the faculty for perceiving affects, and that our language bears traces of this neglect. He refers to our linear memory

aberrant, and man's relations to his surroundings are regarded as a mixture of the tenuous and the arbitrary.[a]

Some students have given their attention directly to the recovery and enlargement of some of the aspects of language that have tended to be submerged under a language of signs. Without minimizing the importance of continuing to develop a language of fixed signs, they have explored ways of enhancing the symbolic possibilities inherent in human language.

Cassirer* has been foremost in contrasting theories of language and of learning based upon response to signs and those which include the complexities of symbolic meaning.[b]

All the phenomena which are commonly described as conditioned reflexes are not merely very far from but even opposed to the essential character of human symbolic thought.[c]

For the sake of a clear statement of the problem we must carefully distinguish between signs and symbols. That we find rather complex systems of signs and signals in animal behavior seems to be an ascertained fact. We may even say that some animals, especially domesticated animals, are extremely susceptible to signs.[d]

A sign or signal is related to the thing to which it refers in a fixed and unique way. Any one concrete and individual sign refers to a certain individual thing.

. . . But this bears no analogy, as it has often been interpreted, to human symbolism; on the contrary, it is in opposition to symbolism. A genuine human symbol is characterized not by its uniformity but by its versatility.[e]

Similarly, Jung distinguishes between sign, an embodiment of a conventionally accepted shorthand, and symbol, the best pos-

for intellectual elements, and our nonlinear memory which has no language for affects. (*The Psychology of Daydreams,* Allen and Unwin, 1921, pp. 25, 189, 209, 201.)

* Jenkins, while recognizing the importance of Cassirer's analysis of language, believes that Cassirer's emphasis on man as a creator of symbols excludes the possibility of discovery of the world outside of man, and segregates man from all outside influences. Much that Cassirer says certainly seems to substitute man for external reality, but development of the symbolic possibilities in language can include discovery as well as creation. What Jenkins says of Cassirer's creating something out of nothing seems to me to apply more to some existentialists than to Cassirer.

sible formulation of a relatively unknown thing, always a creation of a complex nature.[a] In Jung's view the use of symbols helps to bring unconscious creative forces into relation with conscious effort, and the basic biological needs of man into relation with his social world, which lives by shared symbols as well as by more arbitrary and external signs. Jung's distinction between sign and symbol inheres not only in their objective character but in their subjective meaning for the person. The symbol is always complex because both its own human and social history and all facets of the personality of the person employing it enter into its creation and use. Many, but not all, symbols are embodied in concrete images. Whitehead, likewise, stresses the active synthetic role of symbols in expressing relationships "from things to words on the part of the speaker, from words back to things on the part of the listener." [b]

Whatmough takes a somewhat intermediate position between those who advocate a fixed language of signs and those who are interested in the creation of a more complex language of symbols. His first definition of symbol is surrogate, that which substitutes for something else;[c] he is emphatic in saying that language is first and foremost a means of transmitting information;[d] and he repeatedly goes out of his way to denounce Joyce, in particular *Finnegans Wake,* as an attempt at creative symbolism that violates the English language. But he says that it is *fortunate* that language cannot assign as "strictly defined, rigid, and unchanging meaning" to a "symbol" as can logic and mathematics, and that in linguistics identity of meaning is only a convenient fiction.[e] He also regards it as a fault to postulate a direct connection between symbol and referend.[f] He recognizes that neither philosopher nor poet nor scientist dispenses with constructs and that these constructs enter into the formation of symbols,[g] and that both science and poetry require a high degree of creative imagination.[h] But, in a somewhat deprecatory tone, he says that there are experiences "which we cannot yet justify scientifically" and that "imaginative treatment need not be devoid of significance." [i] Whatmough recognizes and appreciates artistic as well as scientific imagination, and in some statements he refers to a symbol as a creation, something more than a surrogate for a phenomenon. But he tends to distrust creative imagination if it goes too far, and to some extent to regard poetry as existing in an intermediate stage until science can take over.

Goldstein, Schilder, Schachtel, and Sullivan are exceptional among psychoanalysts and clinical psychologists in regarding capacity to express thought in multidimensional symbolic language and to engage in abstract thought as fundamental in human nature—as basic as instinctive or libidinal emotional drives. According to this view thought and language are not detours, secondary or substitute devices, because they develop later than, say, the sucking impulse, any more than genital sexuality is a secondary process because it is not fully developed until puberty.

Schilder, Sullivan, and others have observed the infant's awareness of nuances of emotional communication which precedes understanding of the meaning of separate words. "The child 'understands' language before he can use it. An awareness of emotion as expressed in words and an appreciation of the melody of speech precedes the understanding of the content of the words." [a] Psychiatrists who have done extensive work with schizophrenics—Sullivan, Fromm-Reichmann, Sechehaye, Kurt R. Eissler, for example—all stress the sensitivity of the schizophrenic to nonverbalized emotional tones in an interpersonal situation, a sensitivity that has elements in common with the mode of experiencing of infancy and early childhood.

> . . . the infant possesses the faculty of reacting extremely sensitively to emotional changes in the environment . . . the schizophrenic regresses in this respect to a level in which he reacquires a faculty which the nonschizophrenic has lost. . . . His interpretative faculty of emotional . . . manifestations in the external world is sharpened.[b]

Is this range of sensitivity one of the capacities that the fully functioning adult may retain instead of losing it with the acquisition of language? One of the central differences between brain-injured and healthy persons, Goldstein believes, is the difference in their ability to use symbols, which he calls abstract thought. Through abstract thought not only intellectual but emotional experiences and possibilities, otherwise unattainable, become accessible.

> The impairment of the attitude toward the abstract shows in every performance of the brain-damaged patient . . . the patient is unable to deal with a situation which is only possible . . . one may characterize the deficiency as an inability to discover the essence of a situation which is not related to his own personality [or which includes more than the immediate present].[a]

We may quarrel with Goldstein's particular use of abstract and concrete; we may say that he has oversimplified the contrasts.[b] But I do not see how, without lopping off large areas of personality and reality that must be taken into account, we can ignore his insistence on the multidimensional character of healthy human experience and of the importance of the search for a language that can more fully express this character while, at the same time, maintaining its integrity as language.

Korzybski has attempted to find ways of getting beyond the limitations that Aristotelian language forms seem to impose on our habits of perceiving and of thinking, and to discover means of expression in language that will convey a nonelemental, multiordinal view of the world. He contrasts Aristotelian language orientations, which are subject-predicate, either-or, additive linear, elementistic, with new possibilities in language orientations, which are relational, representing flexible degree rather than either-or, non-linear, nonelementistic.[c]

Like Sapir and Whorf, Korzybski stresses the fact that language may not be simply a reflection or even an organization of experience, but is itself, also, "a self-contained, creative symbolic organization," which actually "defines experience for us."[d] He notes that words for the same object may influence our perception by stressing different aspects of that object; the Greek word *men* for the moon stressed its function as a measure of time, whereas the Latin word *luna* stressed its brightness. To some extent at least, we read into the world the structure of the language we use. The world that each of us perceives is not an objective world of happenings, but an object-subject world of happenings and meanings.[a] Lack of recognition of the extent to which language influences perception may decrease objectivity. Development of the symbolic as well as the signaling possibilities in language extends the range of human experience.

As emphasis on a language of signs may constrict the aspects of experience that can find verbal form, so expansion of the symbolic possibilities of language may enlarge the means of communicating shame, the sense of identity, and other diffused experiences, and also of becoming able to apprehend such experiences.

FIVE

The Search for Identity

These reflections began with consideration of the insistence with which the questions Who am I? Where do I belong? press upon us at present, and of the possibility that the self-revealing —and world-revealing—experiences of shame might offer one clue to the discovery of identity. Experiences of shame are a painful uncovering of hitherto unrecognized aspects of one's personality as well as of unrecognized aspects of one's society and of the world. If it is possible to face them, instead of seeking protection from what they reveal, they may throw light on who one is, and hence point the way toward who and what one may become.

Descriptions of some characteristic situations in which shame is felt pointed to the searching nature of these experiences. An account of some of the assumptions and methods of contemporary psychology and social science suggested ways in which these methods tend to place certain limits on understanding of such experiences as shame and identity. Some of the more comprehensive and flexible, although as yet less well-formulated, concepts and methods that are coming into use were presented as possibly leading toward greater understanding.

What follows is an attempt to explore further some of the implications of the preceding chapters. These tentative comments are far from meeting the requirements of theories of the middle-range or intermediate hypotheses.[a] At most, they may perhaps call attention to some underemphasized aspects of familiar phenomena that are relevant to the understanding of identity.

In the most homogeneous society in a relatively tranquil historical period there is no one kind of identity for different individuals, still less any single road leading toward a sense of self and of one's place in society. Even in our more disordered and heterogeneous society, however, we may come a little further in apprehending what attitudes and ways of behaving seem to lead away from, and what ones bring us closer to, discovering who we are.

Inadequate Approaches to Identity

Before suggesting certain kinds of awareness and ways of life that may offer promise of helping to develop a sense of identity I shall mention some contemporary attitudes that seem to me to bypass the problem. Each of these orientations may be for some persons the best way of life. But there is sometimes a tendency to regard each of them more widely as the most desirable life-style possible.

One such attitude, protection of oneself from the exposure of shame before the event, has been mentioned in connection with the difficulty of communicating experiences of shame.* Hazards that may accompany or follow from exposure in the contemporary world increase this impulse for protection. The search for a coherent personality presents special difficulties in a time when the unexpected is continually happening, when the dangers involved in certain kinds of deviation from custom are great, and when it is not easy to know where, or in what or whom, one can put trust. A natural response to this situation is the seeking of some sort of external protection. And this use of external protection may become a depersonalization which takes any one of a number of related forms: adoption of a pose, or of a socially approved role, or adherence to a prescribed

* See pp. 64-70.

right side of a cause.* Each of these forms of externalization offers protection from exposure, but, for some persons at least, at the cost of diminished personal identity.

Protection through depersonalization in the 1920's, particularly in America, appeared in the code of the pose. The pose combined indifference and success. One should at all costs protect oneself from sudden discovery that one was out of perspective, from being ridiculous. The readiest defense against the danger of being ridiculous was to take nothing seriously, and to be nonchalantly successful in the accepted manner in whatever one did. The great word was "amusing"; one should endeavor to be amusing and to find everything else amusing—from Thurber's amusing little Burgundy to the amusing idea of committing suicide. The goal was not significance, but success and a pose of not being earnest. Nothing was free from the success standard. One should be a success in sex, a success in personal relations and in one's profession, an inside dopester in politics—and indifferent to all.

There is a seeming contradiction here in that the 1920's was a period when many people who seemed to make most use of the code of the pose were also those who outdid each other in being ridiculous, outlandish, extravagant, bizarre. But the protection against being thought ridiculous by others might be to act more of a fool than anyone else, to get there first. One could indulge in any extravagance so long as one knew that it was only a pose, never took it seriously. A genuine remark might be quickly followed by the assurance that one was "only kidding." An effort—one's own or another's—to deal thoughtfully with a social issue or a social theory could be brought into line or quickly discounted as a "welcome addition to our light summer reading." If anything seemingly serious can be immediately laughed at as a pose, then one sees around it oneself; it is not ridiculous, not exposure of oneself. Of Amory and Eleanor,

* A particular pose, or role, or belief in a socially approved cause may, of course, coincide with the deepest desires of the individual, in which case it ceases to be depersonalization or external protection. I am speaking of those situations in which the pose or role or adherence to a cause substitutes for or denies personal desire or belief.

F. Scott Fitzgerald says, "Their poses were strewn about the pale dawn like broken glass." In *The Sun Also Rises,* Brett deplores Robert Cohen's desire for significance: "He can't believe it didn't mean anything."

In the 1950's depersonalization appears in the code of the role. The role is distinguished from the pose in part by the recognition it receives, not only, like the pose of the 1920's, in fiction, but in the writings of psychologists and of social scientists. According to some psychologists both the sense of self and the self-ideal approach a "nothing-but" combination of various social roles.[a]

The term role comprises the way others who represent social standards expect an individual to behave, the individual's response to these expectations, and his expectation of approval if he acts in the appropriate manner. These expectations have reference to the positions a person occupies in society as employer, employee, government official, voter, husband, wife, father, mother, child. His social role is what is expected of him by virtue of his place in society, what he responds to, and what he gets for his response. Precise definition of particular social roles is less clear in the contemporary United States than in many other societies, but the combination of lack of clarity in what is expected with insistence that expectation be met can be especially coercive. Acceptance of the concept of roles may come to mean that one acts in a drama that one has had no part in writing or casting; and even sometimes that the psychologist or the social scientist may be cast in the role of director.*

If one rejects the roles prescribed by one's immediate culture in favor of more individual or more widely human values one tends to be alone. This particular kind of aloneness is, as noted above, the theme of many contemporary novels. It is the problem of the protagonist in *The Strong Box.*

> If confided in as to the strongbox letters . . . more than one of his colleagues would listen with intelligent sympathy and begin, Well, of course you're best out, as I see it. And if you replied that you did not want out but rather felt a responsibility to stay in, he would say, Oh in that case it's a personal matter and you have to judge for

* David Riesman has suggested this formulation.

yourself. And the inference would plainly be that most successful men in New York never involved themselves in personal matters.[a]

The same theme is developed in the novels of C. P. Snow in England. Edith Weigert has pointed out the way in which the tendency to expect that persons will meet and "take" each other in a variety of roles that represent what they are supposed to be by virtue of their place in society may block the discovery of who they are as individual human beings.*

In some situations the destruction of personal identity and personal relations to make way for a particular social role is deliberate on the part of a particular group in society, and may be also a deliberate choice on the part of the individuals whose identity is destroyed and replaced by a role. The training of an American army officer is described by a psychologist who observed the process in an Officer Candidate School in the Second World War.

The practices start with the assumption that . . . candidates are highly motivated to become officers. The hopeful candidate is . . . subjected to a nearly catastrophic experience, which breaks down to a large extent his previous personality organization. His previous valuations fail him and in order to find a basis for self-respect, he must adopt new standards or escape from the field.

Progressive identification with the officer role is most adequately fostered in schools which have graded classes in various stages of training. . . . The "gigging" and personal degradation of the lower-class man become tolerable to him when he sees them as a necessary condition for . . . a status position he himself will some day occupy. The personal indignity of the lower-class man . . . is thus established for him as one of the status rewards of the position toward which he is climbing.

An additional mechanism . . . in the determination of the officer personality is the passing-on of aggression. As a lower-class man . . . the would-be officer cannot respond with aggression to the affronts of upper-class men and officers in general. . . . This fund of repressed aggression is one of the features of the ordeal contributing to personality disorganization. . . . His ego is impoverished by inwardly directed aggressive trends. To feel himself a man again . . . he seeks aggressively to assert his superiority over someone else.[b]

* Cf. p. 154.

This sort of destruction of identity and of feeling for other persons is defended by many military officers as a necessity for military training. The extent to which it is a necessity was hotly debated in the controversy arising out of the drowning of six marines in a disciplinary march at Parris Island.

> The old philosophy of how to make a Marine at Parris Island was not unlike that of brainwashing—a term, but not an idea, born in Korea.
>
> It was to tear apart the youth that came [as a recruit], destroying every shred of his personality and individuality, and then to build him back up again into a stereotyped, emotionless, disciplined fighting machine.
>
> . . . the base training officer, says the theory here is still the same —"but we don't tear them down so far."
>
> Today . . . [the recruit] is still disciplined, but he retains his personality.
>
> The men who leave . . . [under the revised regulations] are probably in better physical shape than ever before. But whether they are men emotionally ready for their job as professional killers is debated. And whether all the abuse can ever be eliminated is questioned.[a]

The implications for individuals and for society of replacing personal identity by a military role become more important as military preparation becomes a larger part of national planning. A number of searching questions are raised by the Parris Island incident: Can a training officer justly be punished for exercising exactly those traits he has been trained to develop? Can one act toward other human beings as something less than human when they are labeled "enemies" and not act in the same way in other situations toward human beings not so labeled? Can dehumanized attitudes toward other persons be developed in the military institutions of a society without spreading to other areas of the society?

This last question is relevant to the analysis by a Harvard economist of American capitalism in a manner that leads to debate as to whether he is being simply matter-of-fact or ironic. He describes the impact of the Second World War on the United States.

For the great majority of Americans World War II . . . was an almost casual and pleasant experience. Several million found jobs who had doubted whether they might ever find jobs again. Hundreds of thousands of others escaped the routine of middle-class employments, their boredom with which they had concealed even from themselves. . . . Only a minority experienced *the nagging homesickness, the fear, the physical suffering and the mutilation and death* which is *the less pleasant destiny* of the fighting soldier in wartime. Because they were a minority the war left no lasting imprint.[a] (Italics mine.)

Questions involved in the substitution of prescribed social roles for individual identity—for example, the values of business organization for personal idiom—are relevant also to the values of the suburbanites that William H. Whyte, Jr., describes as substitutes for any inner aspects of personality development.[b] Potential leaders in the suburbanite culture tend to equate the desire of an individual to be alone with psychic disorder; ". . . the basis of the Social Ethic is not conformity but a sense of moral imperative." [c] "Most [of the younger generation] see themselves as objects more acted upon than acting . . . determined as much by the system as by themselves." [d] "To preach . . . the skills of getting along isolated from why and to what end the getting along is for does not produce maturity. . . . It is easy to fight obvious tyranny; it is not easy to fight benevolence, and few things are more calculated to rob the individual of his defenses than the idea that his interests and those of society can be wholly compatible . . . one who lets The Organization be the judge ultimately sacrifices himself." [e]

A special version of protection from vulnerability through the adoption of correct social roles and correct social attitudes appears in the United States. For Americans, as for all other peoples, a generalized concept of national character is a great oversimplification. But it is nevertheless true that certain ways of feeling and behaving tend to distinguish inhabitants of the United States, in many sections of the country, from other peoples. One of these is a tendency to believe that to every problem there is a here-and-now right or best answer, and that if one acts in terms of the right answer one's efforts should meet with success.[a] This belief provides a basis for the optimism so valued by Americans.*

This kind of emphasis on "right" answers is, as Margaret Mead has observed, a special, by no means a universal, cultural characteristic. ". . . this type of character in which the individual is reared to ask first not 'Do I want it?' or 'Am I afraid?' or 'Is this the custom?' but 'Is this right or wrong?'—is a very special development, characteristic of our own culture, and of a very few other societies." [b] How many American children in the last fifty years have been brought up on the precept "There is a right way and a wrong way to do everything, and you might just as well learn the right way as the wrong way." † So deeply ingrained among certain groups in our society is the habit of looking always for what ought to be done that it is hard for children to phrase their desires in any other way. This is perhaps particularly true of children brought up in families that combine a strong religious background with limited economic circumstances, and it was probably truer of children in the early part of the century than at present. But this way of thought has not disappeared, and we still hear children of financially modest, conscientious parents saying not that "It might be fun" to do something but: "It's a nice day. We ought to have a picnic." "There is time before supper. We ought to go swimming." "I have no homework. I ought to watch television." Some children classify their toys and their books as "information" and "fun." This manner of speaking seems to arise from a necessity to fit everything into an accepted code and an inability to express desire without moral sanction. Moreover, this attitude often carries within it the unstated assumption that right action should be rewarded.

The expectation of favorable outcome of right action applies to public as well as to private life. Americans find it hard to believe that if we work hard and do right we will not attain our

* Discussions in the 1956 Presidential election of the dangers of atomic warfare were condemned by many people as "pessimistic."

† The term right carried a Platonic mingling of what is functionally efficient and what is morally good.

aims. Since success is regarded as the reward of merit, if in complex domestic or foreign affairs we do not attain what we want, we tend to ask, Whose fault is it? Insurance companies ask about an automobile accident, not What caused it? but Whose fault was it? If China becomes Communist we do not study the history of China; we ask through whose villainy we "lost" China. Before Sputnik, if the Soviet Union developed atomic energy, we did not study the development of Soviet science, we asked who gave away our secrets. We gave money to Europe; we sent the largest number of troops to Korea; if things still don't come out right, there must be a villain somewhere. We tend to line up on one side of an issue or a cause and to feel that we have lost our identity if we can't be sure that we are on the side of the right. It is hard for a people accustomed to believe that an immediate right answer can be discovered in any situation and who have little in the artifacts of daily life to remind them of long historical processes to realize the extent to which history not only opens possibilities but also sets limits on right answers. Yet in some situations a "right" anwer can be discovered only in the course of historical processes that extend over a long period of time, and unless we realize this we may make even more difficult any answer to the question Where do I belong?

Protection from vulnerability through depersonalization, by the adoption of socially approved poses or roles or right answers to issues, tends to be a nothing-but view of alternative positions. If you have tensions, learn how to release tensions. If you have been emotionally hurt, reduce your emotions. If some people in our society are unsuccessful, show them how to adopt the appropriate roles and attitudes to achieve prestige and success. The imperative of daily living is "get out of my way so that I can take your place." [a] Success in a role means prestige; failure means shame.

These external protective devices, while they may seem to give security through status and avoid risk of exposure and being found ridiculous—making the discovery of identity unnecessary or dulling the sense of need for it—may actually for some persons intensify the need.[b] There may come for them a horror at finding the pose or the role the only thing left, sex arid, success meaningless. Avoidance of personal encounter and commitment may result in feeling that persons cease to be human, that nothing makes any difference, and eventually that nothing is real.

The aridity that may be the outcome of attempts at protection through externalization and depersonalization appears in some writers who are among the most articulate in interpreting the contemporary world and are themselves most representative of some aspects of it. Dislike for and distrust of human beings and disparagement of any serious encounter they may have with each other and with their society appears in writers as different as Aldous Huxley, Ernest Hemingway, W. H. Auden, and Arthur Koestler. Moreover, this human detachment increases in the course of their writings.

Of Huxley, Edmund Wilson says: "Merely a manipulator of Punch-and-Judy figures, he . . . has to shake them off his hands and to use these hands in pulpit gestures as he comes forward to preach his way of life . . . his readiness to reject the world is due to his not knowing what is in it . . . he . . . never had the full sense of what humanity was like and, hence, of what it might become. . . . Huxley's satire has always been founded . . . upon a distaste for humanity." [a] In the course of Hemingway's writing Wilson has traced a similar insulation of his characters, an increasing loss of interest in human beings, a growing tendency to drug, rather than to express, disquieting emotions.[b] Pritchett believes that he sees the same process of the sharpening of the intellect and style and the impoverishment of emotion in Auden.[c] Lionel Trilling finds as characteristic of contemporary fiction writers in the *New Yorker* a similar disbelief in life, exploitation of the unwariness of characters, and a desire for moral grandeur "at small emotional expense." [d] With each successive novel and with each section of his autobiography, Koestler shows more distrust of people and of political beliefs they may hold. He rejects, not only his own former belief in communism, but any aspiration that might lead to active political engagement. He diverts attention from the human situation that was supposedly at one time his main concern to his own sentiments.*

External protection from risks of exposure through various forms of depersonalization may, as the work of both Huxley and Koestler shows, extend itself into its opposite: an emphasis on inner life which denies all importance to social participation, and exalts contemplation *over against* action. Some forms of existentialism represent this sort of disavowal of any possible meaning in social identifications and in social action.

A similar disparagement of action and of relations to other persons as compared with one's own inner feeling appears in certain literary circles. Malcolm Cowley has described this preoccupation in a review of studies in modern European literature:

> . . . who are the modern authors, and what are the qualities that make them modern? . . . Baudelaire . . . was born in 1821 and thus was only about ten years younger than Tennyson, Thackeray, Dickens and Browning. . . . Why do we call him a modern while dismissing the others as early Victorian?
>
> . . . The four Englishmen . . . reflected the ideals of an apparently stable society, whereas Baudelaire stood apart from society and tried to express his own troubled and unhappy heart. He was modern . . . by the nervous intensity of his emotions and by their unconventional nature . . . by the cool, ironical, almost scientific fashion in which he observed the emotions, and by the defiant honesty with which he revealed them.
>
> Using Baudelaire as a touchstone, we can decide which European authors are modern in this particular meaning of the word. . . . They would be authors who stood apart from business or politics and lived in an inner world of emotions, so that "subjective" is a key word applied to them.[a]

Is it characteristic of some contemporaries that it is more tolerable to believe that the world holds no meaning than that they as individuals have failed? Sartre, Camus, and others have

* Koestler's latest book, *Reflections on Hanging* (Macmillan, 1957), although concerned with a social issue, does not seem to me to represent an essentially different trend in his thought.

created a community of isolated men in which the universe is shamed but the individuals maintain dignity and a—paradoxical—sense of being together. One is related to others by a sharing of alienation.

Search for identity by withdrawal, by accent on personal, rather than on social or political concerns, has been strengthened by reaction to the political disappointments that followed the 1930's. It can lead, as in some forms of existentialism, to a concentration on tragedy as the only significant human experience and to an identification of particular social and historical limitations with the limitations of man's fate.

As the awareness of the self grows with the growing awareness of the external world and with the delineation of the self as distinct from other realities, so, as belief in the importance of the real world diminishes, full confrontation of the self may also diminish. This has been true of Koestler as of others who have sought to escape the difficulties of the present human situation by turning their backs on it. There results a preoccupation with personal feeling—in which even that is lost. This depersonalization, extending to dehumanization, can become a negative counterpart of identity.

It might be mentioned, parenthetically, that another form of the extension of externalization into its opposite is an appeal for a return to reason which turns out to be a disguised exhortation to return to a particular tradition. Max Horkheimer, for example, believes that what he regards as the current eclipse of reason should be overcome by a revival of Hegelian and Marxian thought.[a] For T. S. Eliot (as for Reinhold Niebuhr) restoration of reason demands a revival of religious faith and a sense of sin. Neither the Marxist Horkheimer nor the Anglo-Catholic Eliot fully faces the fact that it is not enough to assume that any one tradition, however rich and however honored, is synonymous with reason, but that whatever the tradition we regard as most fruitful, we cannot escape the responsibility of interpretation and selection.

For many Americans neither the religious tradition invoked by Eliot nor the philosophical tradition of Horkheimer has great appeal. It is the tradition of democratic liberalism that seems to them reasonable, self-explanatory, and self-justifying. The reiteration of nineteenth-century liberalism or Jeffersonian democracy may lead them to think that they can, in Pritchett's words, continue to live "on the easy capital of the enlightenment." The implications of the kind of individualism that can be realized only through recognition of intermeshing social relationships and an adequate twentieth-century interpretation of Marxian theory are still to be developed.

Special Importance and Difficulties of Psychoanalysis

Psychoanalytic theory and psychoanalytic therapy stand in a special relation to the search for identity.* Psychoanalysis is of all professions the one most avowedly and directly concerned with the discovery of identity. It would be impossible to explore the meaning of shame and of identity without special reference to psychoanalysis. My special indebtedness to Erikson, Schachtel, Schilder, Sullivan, and other psychoanalysts has appeared throughout this discussion. I shall speak in more detail below of Erikson's study of identity.

Just because of the strategic position of psychoanalysis in relation to identity, however, and because of the position of psychoanalysis in contemporary American thought, it is necessary to speak of the particular anomalies and hazards of the profession. This is a difficult subject to discuss, in part because judgment about it tends to be submerged under the vehemence and in-group thinking of its supporters (and even of supporters of particular schools) and the equal vehemence of its critics, and also because one's own emotional involvements, though they enter into any appraisal, are particularly concerned in the appraisal of psychoanalysis. But psychoanalysis is a phenom-

* Psychoanalytic theory and therapy cannot, I think, validly be separated as much as is sometimes done. Freud's theory grew directly from his observations in therapy and was continually modified by further observations. The way therapy is conducted is in turn modified in the light of changes in the theory. What appears in the free associations and in the dreams of patients in treatment, as well as the disappearance of symptoms, is frequently cited as proof of the rightness of the theory.

enon of the contemporary world, and we must try to appraise it. Five hundred years from now it may be appraised very differently, but we must do what we can with the knowledge we have.

No profession has ever occupied a position or assumed a responsibility entirely comparable to that of psychoanalysis. The psychoanalyst has been compared to a surgeon. But because of the kind of intimate relation he has and encourages with his patient, his own character and his personal values enter into his therapeutic methods in a way and to an extent that is not true for the surgeon. He has been compared to a priest. But the priest by the nature of his assumptions does not do the kind of detailed probing over a period of years that the analyst does; and, to many persons who seek psychoanalysis today, to speak with the voice of Science is more than to speak with the voice of God. This particular combination of intimacy and impersonal authority is, I think, without precedent. It gives to the analyst enormous power. The persons who come to him are vulnerable, and the process of analysis tends, at least in its initial stages, to increase their vulnerability. Both because of the methods they use and the content of their therapy, there is probably no group of persons today—with the exception of priests and some practitioners of "mental healing"—in a position to exercise as much power over persons with whom they come into professional contact as psychoanalysts. This power aims to be, and often is, a means of bringing to the individual seeking treatment greater freedom and fuller realization of himself. But it can achieve this aim only if the psychoanalyst recognizes the extent of his power and of its hazards. Freud clearly recognized this power and its hazards (as well as the difficulties involved in "counter-transference"), and emphasis on such recognition is increasingly a part of training in psychoanalysis.

There would seem to be two situations in which the kind of opening of oneself that is an essential of the analytic treatment is possible: one where the relation is one of mutuality, and there is in trust and love the opening of two persons to each other; the other where the person to whom one opens oneself is the surrogate of God or of some higher power. The analyst is in neither of these situations; he is likely to stand first on one foot, then on the other, and few analysts seem to me to have confronted the full complexity of this problem. Sullivan insisted on the importance of mutuality and communication; but the analyst does not open himself to the patient as the patient is expected to do to the analyst. Freud and the early Freudians leaned toward the conception of the remote analyst, an embodiment of a higher wisdom; but no analyst, however skillful and however humane, is all-wise and all-good. The late Frieda Fromm-Reichmann[a] seems to me to have come nearest to seeing this problem in its full dimensions. She carried to amazing lengths the ability to be open to the patient, to adapt to his views, to see the world through his eyes, but she was quite clear that the analyst remains the expert; the relation is not, and cannot be, one of mutuality.

In the attempt to appraise psychoanalysis there must be consideration of both method and content: the method of psychoanalysis, the assumptions involved in the relation between analyst and patient, and the content of analysis—what a particular school of psychoanalytic thought or a particular analyst considers a desirable outcome of therapy. The general aim of the analyst—sometimes more fully, sometimes less fully, achieved—is to help the patient to be more secure and happy in the realization of his own identity, or at least to remove neurotic obstacles to such realization.

But the achievement of this aim through the methods of psychoanalysis involves the deliberate breaking down of one identity and replacing it by another, accomplishing this in part through the "transference" of the patient to the analyst and "overcoming the resistance" of the patient to the analyst's implicit or explicit ideas of what is desirable, healthy, mature, and realistic. Ruth Munroe reports that the aim of psychoanalysis "is fundamental change in the personality," to establish firmly "a basic shift in attitude." [b] If this is true, then the psychoanalytic process would seem to have something in common with the substitution of one personality for another in military training described above, and with religious and political conversion. The analyst, of course, always attempts to make the new identity that replaces the old what the patient "really" wants, just as the religious or political leader says that he is expressing the "real" wishes of the people. These interpretations may be valid. But, as in any human relation—teaching, therapy, political or religious leadership, or any other—complete "objectivity" is impossible and the values of the interpreter enter into the interpretation.

The similarity in these different processes of changing identity and the problems this presents is recognized by students most sympathetic to psychoanalysis and by psychoanalysts themselves. Joost A. M. Meerloo, a Dutch psychoanalyst now in the United States, in a study of methods of totalitarian mass coercion,[a] has pointed out that mental coercion is more effective than physical torture in breaking down personality;[b] that just as educational training can degenerate into coercive training, so therapy can degenerate into the imposition of the doctor's will on the patient;[c] and that since a psychological interview is in itself a coercive situation, the therapist must use enormous care and restraint not to exert his influence unduly.[d] He believes that psychoanalysts recently have become more aware of these problems and have taken greater care to avoid them.

One of the most arresting recent studies of the methods of psychoanalysis is that of William Sargant, President of the Section of Psychiatry of the British Royal Society of Medicine.[e] Using as a basis for comparison the experiments of Pavlov in inducing neuroses in dogs, he examines in detail what he believes to be the common physiological and psychological processes involved in psychoanalysis and in methods of destroying political and religious beliefs which are of the essence of a person's identity, and of replacing them by others.[f] Sargant begins his foreword by saying that he is discussing only *methods* of changing personality, *not* the nature of the changes or the content of the beliefs imparted. "It must be emphasized as strongly as possible that this book is *not* concerned with the truth or falsity of any particular religious or political belief. Its purpose is to examine some of the mechanisms involved in the fixing or destroying of such beliefs in the human brain."

Sargant's analysis is, I think, open to question on a number of grounds: Granted that there may be common physiological and psychological factors involved in the different processes he describes, differences are more important than he indicates. Under extreme pressure almost every individual may have an ultimate breaking point, where he abandons "resistance" and human reason and becomes indistinguishable from a salivating dog,[a] but it makes a great difference where this point comes.* One thing that helps to determine the degree of resistance to pressure—the previous experience of the person—is more important than Sargant seems to recognize. A person who has never known poverty, social frustration, or injustice may be less receptive to Communist doctrines; a person who has not experienced a sense of sin and of the futility of earthly life, to the religious evangelist; a person who has not felt himself hampered by conflict and inability to direct his own life, to psychoanalytic interpretations. Sargant also underestimates the enormous differences between the psychological processes that are involved if a person has voluntarily sought out the Communist party or the church or the psychoanalyst or military training and those involved if he involuntarily finds himself in the concentration camp or in the army. Furthermore, the character and content of the beliefs and identity destroyed and those that replace them seem to me to be far more important in relation to the methods used than Sargant allows.

But with all these serious qualifications, the similarities in the experiences of psychoanalysis and of religious and political conversion are phenomena that no one interested in the theoretical and therapeutic possibilities of psychoanalysis can ignore. Examining these similarities is not equating psychoanalysis with religious or political conversion. It is simply saying that certain processes in some respects similar are involved in these different experiences, and that these similarities merit examination by anyone interested in the possibilities of psychoanalysis for increasing human freedom.

Sargant points out that in the initial stages of psychoanalysis,

* All that has been said earlier of the fallacies of applying animal experiments to human beings applies to Sargant's analysis.

as of political and religious conversion, anxiety, humiliation, and guilt are increased—often augmented by physical fatigue and debility resulting from the anxiety aroused by the process itself—so that the patient becomes more and more dependent on the analyst.[a] "As the analysis proceeds, and emotional storms mount" these "transference situations" are built up so that the patient becomes increasingly sensitized to suggestions that he would earlier have rejected. Sargant gives illustrations of persons who dream dreams that conform to the doctrine of a particular analyst, and even of the same person dreaming dreams that differ according to the doctrines of successive analysts of different schools of psychoanalysis.[b] After abreactions* over a period of months or even years the therapist may be able to bring about changes in the patient's ideas and behavior without too much difficulty;[c] the patient "will sometimes 'box the compass' in his views on religion or politics, or in his attitude to his family and friends." [d]

A stage is finally reached "when resistance weakens to the therapist's interpretations of a patient's symptoms. . . . He now believes and acts upon theories about his nervous condition which, more often than not, contradict his former beliefs. . . . These changes are consolidated by making [his] behavior as consistent as possible with the new 'insight' gained." "Analysis is often considered complete only when the therapist's points of view have been thoroughly absorbed and resistance . . . to the therapist's interpretations of past events has broken down." [e]

Sargant says that terror and shame play a large part in "being re-made" in therapy, brainwashing, and conversion, that a person particularly responsive to other pressures† is also particularly responsive to analytic pressure[f] and (as Munroe and others have also said) that what is actually involved is the breaking down of one identity and replacing it by one that the analyst,

* Abreaction is defined by Sargant, following W. S. Sadler, as "a process of reviving the memory of a repressed unpleasant experience and expressing in speech and action the emotions related to it, thereby relieving the personality of its influence." (*Battle for the Mind*, Heinemann, 1957, p. 42.)

† Here, I think, he does not sufficiently distinguish among the *kinds of* pressures to which an individual has been responsive in his previous history.

on the basis of the patient's revelations, considers more desirable.

Important as it is to recognize the similarities that Sargant points out, it is also important, as I said above, to recognize the differences in these processes to which Sargant does not give adequate weight: the crucial difference between whether a person voluntarily seeks a change of identity or is forced into a situation that demands it; the variations in susceptibilities to pressure that result from previous life experiences; the content of the new identity considered desirable by the analyst and acceptable to the patient and its relation to these previous experiences of the person engaging in the change.

In regard to the content of psychoanalysis, analysts vary greatly in the extent to which they think that the changed personality that should be the outcome of therapy should embody adjustment to the norms of achievement and success that are the "reality" of contemporary society. For some, ego development turns out to be adaptation to present social norms. For others, the aim of analysis is helping the patient to develop the courage to deviate in his own way from accepted norms.

Fromm, Horney, and to some extent Sullivan take specific issue with some of these accepted norms. They, however, may underestimate the difficulties involved if, on the one hand, the repressions of contemporary society are as great as they say and, on the other, the individual is deemed unworthy if, in spite of these repressions, he is not an independent, productive, mature person. They urge the individual to "be himself" instead of cherishing an unrealistic, ideal self-image or following the dictates of custom and of authority; to have faith, but to make sure that it is a rational faith; in the midst of social coercions to discover his true self.

Fromm, like Goldstein, is chiefly concerned with the self-actualizing possibilities of human beings. In his view the chief threat to realization of identity lies in submission to irrational authority. He believes that, contrary to Freud's view, love and hate have different roots in the personality, and that, contrary to Calvin's view, self-love and love of others are necessarily complementary, not antagonistic. He deplores the "market-place psychology" that dominates contemporary life.

For Fromm the chief terror is isolation, the chief sin is self-mutilation, the chief virtue is spontaneous realization of individual potentialities through productive work and productive relations with others.[a] But what is this real, spontaneous self independent of romanticism and of all authority—or at least of all irrational authority—that we are exhorted to realize? If the psychology of the market place, of achievement, and of success are to be repudiated, what is the reality that we must accept and adjust to if we are to avoid the unrealities of sentimentality and insubstantial idealism? The difficulties of self-realization in the midst of these conflicts may be more profound than Fromm sometimes seems to recognize.

Marcuse is, I think, too sweeping in his condemnation of Fromm, Horney, and Sullivan as Freudian revisionists; and he does not discuss Fromm's recent book *The Sane Society,* which does precisely question the extent to which it is possible for individuals to achieve productivity and self-realization in capitalist, bourgeois society. Marcuse denounces the revisionist movement because in it, he believes, the regressive features of psychoanalysis have become dominant;[b] therapy is a course in resignation;[c] there is a commitment to this present capitalist society;[d] the individual is held to be personally responsible for failure of self-realization, a view that minimizes the role of society;[e] and the brute fact of social repression is transformed into a moral problem for the individual.*

But admonitions to be one's spontaneous, real self and at the same time to accept reality minimize the difficulties of the problems involved. Learning when to yield to a recalcitrant reality and when to try to change it is a main problem of life,

* Marcuse's basic criticism of the Freudian revisionists is essentially the same as his criticism of the existentialists that "Behind the nihilistic language of the existentialists lurks the ideology of free competition, free initiative, and equal opportunity. Everybody can 'transcend' his situation, carry out his own project. Everybody has his absolutely free choice . . . in Sartre's philosophy . . . 'Pour-soi' vacillates between . . . individual subject and . . . universal Ego or consciousness. Most of the qualities which he attributes to the 'Pour-soi' are qualities of man as a genus . . . *not* the essential qualities of man's concrete existence." ("Existentialism: Remarks on Jean-Paul Sartre's *L'Etre ET LE NEANT," Philosophy and Phenomenological Research,* Vol. VIII, No. 3, Mar. 1948, pp. 323 and 334-5.)

one that must constantly be resolved afresh. The question is not whether to adjust to or to rebel against reality, but, rather, how to discriminate between those realities that must be recognized as unalterable and those that we should continue to try to change however unyielding they may appear. Our whole life is spent in an attempt to discover when our refusal to bow to limitations is romantic escape from actualities and when it is courage and rational faith. There were many who argued that acceptance of reality when Hitler came to power demanded adjustment to Nazism, and that any other action was romantic folly. There are many, among their number psychoanalysts, who argue that being efficient in terms of the money and success values of our achievement society is one of the requirements for realistic mature living. Working for peace or for any form of shared welfare or noncompetitive community life, or for socialism is condemned by some persons as unrealistic sentimentality. And yet—innovation of any sort, in the physical or in the social world, has always been regarded as ridiculous, as unrealistic romanticism. "The idea seems ridiculous, but I can find nothing wrong with it," said Kepler of his concept of infinity. Only the refusal to bow to accepted realities can bring new knowledge of the physical or the psychological world or a new stage of history.

So, too, our whole life is an attempt to discover when our spontaneity is whimsical, sentimental irresponsibility and when it is a valid expression of our deepest desires and values. Horney, Fromm, and even Sullivan at times, seem to assume that there is an already existent real or true or spontaneous self which can be evoked into active existence almost at will. There is a tacit assumption that somehow we know the dictates of the real self, and that we should live in terms of these rather than of a romanticized self-image or of the pseudo-self of others' expectations. But, like understanding of "reality," such a real self is something to be discovered and created, not a given, but a lifelong endeavor.

Marcuse condemns our present society—in terms as far-reaching but less specific than Fromm's; he believes that only a revolution on Marxian lines would be of any use in creating a more humane social order and that individuals cannot hope to escape the repressions of this society. But Marcuse, Fromm, and any social scientist who believes that a society more expressive of individual desires is a possibility must confront the question of how we get from here to there. They must recognize, as Marx did, that some individuals are freer than others from the coercions of their class and their historical situation and can therefore take a more aware and active part than the majority in the historical processes that shape the future.

Erikson's Concept of Identity and the Guilt-Axis and Shame-Axis Approaches to Identity

Erikson's explicit recognition of the present importance of the problem of identity was quoted earlier.* I shall here describe in more detail his hypotheses related to the meaning and conditions of the discovery of identity, and then go on to discuss the implications inherent in and the questions raised by his, Schachtel's, and similar formulations.

In using the word identity, instead of self or ego or any of their variations, Erikson deliberately selects a term that has a double direction, that clearly indicates that some sort of correspondence between the inner and the outer world is indispensable for a sense of identity. He uses the term identity with multiple connotations, which include: unconscious and conscious strivings for continuity of personality, a tendency toward synthesis beyond even unconscious striving, a criterion for the outcome of this striving and this tendency, a maintenance of congruence with the ideals and identity of one's social group, a conscious awareness of who one is.[a] By implication he includes in the meaning of identity the self as subject and as object, as observer and observed—meanings that are sometimes kept separate in an effort to make exclusive distinctions between the concepts self and ego.

This ambiguity, this multidimensional character, of the term identity is not, I believe, a drawback in its use.[b] We may

* See p. 14.

question a particular connotation Erikson gives to the term and still recognize that its very ambiguity, the surplus meaning it carries, makes it more accurately descriptive of the awareness of "I" that may emerge from the processes of integrating life experiences than the narrower conceptions of self and ego. In part because of his very use of the double-directed term identity Erikson seems to me to make a special contribution to the understanding of the way in which the various identifications and introjections of the developing individual are woven into the "I" and the "me." In his view the integration into the "I" is more than a sum or an integration of social roles, more than the *persona,* although these are parts of the fabric.

Erikson regards the awareness of identity as a special characteristic of one stage of development and also as essential for maturity. He traces eight stages in the development of personality, each of which involves a conflict and a possible crisis. Each stage may give rise to special difficulties if its particular conflict is not resolved in a way that is constructive for the growing person, and each has special possibilities for enlargement of personality and increased strength of identity if it is so resolved.[a] Erikson's hypothetical stages of development are important in that they go beyond Gesell's theories of chronological maturation and Freud's theories of sexual phases of growth to explicit recognition of the importance of shifting social relations, and also of greater surplus energy in each stage.

In setting out this pattern of development, Erikson is careful to say that these different stages, and the possible crises and the potentialities for development each presents, are suggested formulations rather than given or proved entities. "I am going to propose a list of these criteria [of ego strength at various stages of development] without knowing exactly what psychological units we are dealing with." [b]

Each potential component strength of developing personality reaches its particular unique ascendancy in one of these stages of conflict and has its own particular vulnerability and possibility at that period. But none of these potential component strengths begins or ends in its period of special climax. Each begins potentially in some form at the beginning of life, and the resolution of conflict that each has found continues in some form throughout life.[a] Each conflict stage is conceived not only, as in the compensatory theory of personality, as a threat of a destructive crisis that must be coped with or overcome, but also as an opportunity for accrued strength.[b] Each stage involves both the inner self and its relation to the social situation in the outer world.

The characteristic conflicts of the eight hypothetical stages of development are:[c] trust vs. mistrust; autonomy vs. shame, doubt;* initiative vs. guilt; industry vs. inferiority; identity vs. identity diffusion; intimacy vs. isolation; generativity (the interest in establishing and guiding the next generation) vs. self-absorption; integrity vs. disgust, despair.†

Erikson regards these eight stages of development as supplementing, not replacing, Freud's theory of periods of development with its emphasis on sexual conflicts and maturation. In the diagrammatic presentation of his eight stages he relates them both to chronological age and to Freud's developmental stages. But he does point out the contrast between the stress in Freudian theory on typical danger situations and his own emphasis on maturation of function, between the Freudian view of the central importance of psychosexual development and his own view of the significance of psychosocial development.[d] At each stage of the developing personality, Erikson believes, there is an access of surplus internal energy and the possibility of enhanced support from social relations that makes it possible for the individual to meet the potential crisis in such a way as to incorporate the resolved conflict into a strengthened identity.

* In this stage the child learns to delineate the area over which he has control and to develop self-esteem. It is the task of society to "back the child up" in his wish to "stand on his own feet" lest he be overcome by the sense of having "gone too far" (shame) or exposed to the mistrust of looking backward (doubt). ("Growth and Crises of the 'Healthy Personality,'" in Clyde Kluckhohn and Henry A. Murray, *Personality in Nature, Society, and Culture,* 2d ed., Knopf, 1953, pp. 199-200.)

† Some statements of Erikson's might lead one to think that he regarded these stages of development as completed at adolescence. Elsewhere, however, he makes it clear that he regards the development of identity as something that continues, at least for some persons, throughout life.

Since each component of the personality exists in some form, latent or overt, at each stage, it would be theoretically possible, according to Erikson, to trace through each stage its components of shame and developing identity. Identity includes, but is more than, what Erikson calls autonomy, since autonomy does not have the double direction of identity.

This tentative formulation of Erikson's which contrasts shame (and doubt of oneself) with autonomy as a stage of growth preceding the conflict of guilt with initiative is relevant to the question of the guilt axis and the shame axis in personality, and of the part each plays in the development of identity. From Erikson's analysis it would follow that shame and guilt are two distinguishable—although not *opposite*—experiences which may at times be linked together, but are not always so linked. Shame, which at least in our culture is often related to visual exposure (including sexual exposure), characteristically occurs, he believes, as an earlier experience than guilt, which is more often related to specific auditory admonition against violation of a code. Shame is doubt, including diffused anxiety, an over-all ashamedness, a consciousness of the whole self, a feeling that life is happening to the individual.[a] Anxiety is peculiarly associated with shame. In every potential crisis of development anxiety is possible, and each new conflict may revive latent anxiety. But anxiety has special relation to the conflict between shame and doubt and the developing sense of what he here calls autonomy. It is not fear, nor anxiety faced directly, but unconfronted aimless anxiety that drives an individual into irrational action, irrational flight—or, indeed, irrational denial of danger.[b]

Guilt, in contrast to shame, is more related to specific acts, going against specific taboos. Basic trust in one's world and especially in the persons who are its interpreters is crucial to one's sense of identity. In shame there is a doubt, a questioning of trust. It is for such reasons as these that shame may be said to go deeper than guilt; it is worse to be inferior and isolated than to be wrong, to be outcast in one's own eyes than to be condemned by society.

The following comparison simply brings together some of

the differences between the guilt axis and the shame axis in personality that have been noted earlier. They are in no sense polar opposites. Both the guilt axis and the shame axis enter into the attitudes and behavior of most people, and often into the same situation. But there are for different persons different balances and stresses between the two, and it does matter whether one lives more in terms of one or of the other. The particular comparisons listed are only suggestive; no two persons would experience these contrasts in exactly the same way. The differences are presented in this way only for the sake of comparison; in experience shame and guilt are usually not so sharply separated.

Guilt Axis	*Shame Axis*
Concerned with each separate, discrete act	Concerned with the over-all self
Involves transgression of a specific code, violation of a specific taboo	Involves falling short, failure to reach an ideal
Involves an additive process; advance to healthy personality by deleting wrong acts and substituting right ones for them	Involves a total response that includes insight, something more than can be reached by addition
Involves competition, measurement on a scale, performing the acts prescribed as desirable	Involves acting in terms of the pervasive qualitative demands of oneself, more rigorous than external codes; each act partakes of the quality of the whole
Exposure of a specific misdemeanor, with emphasis on to whom exposed; exposure of something that should be hidden in a closet	Exposure of the quick of the self, most of all to oneself; exposure of something that can never be hidden in a closet, is in the depths of the earth or in the open sunlight
Concern about violation of social codes of cleanliness, politeness, and so on	Concern about unalterable features of one's body, way of moving, clumsiness, and so on

Guilt Axis—Continued	*Shame Axis—Continued*
Feeling of wrongdoing for a specific harmful act toward someone one loves	Feeling that one may have loved the wrong person, or may be inadequate for the person one loves
Being a good, loyal friend, husband, wife, parent	Having an overflowing feeling for friend, husband, wife, children which makes goodness and loyalty a part of the whole experience with no need for separate emphasis
Trust built on the conception of no betrayal, no disloyal act, as a preliminary to giving affection	Trust that is a process of discovery which gradually eliminates fear of exposure, which is not the result of an act of will but unfolds with the unfolding experience
Feelings of anger, jealousy, meanness for certain socially recognized causes	Inwardly deep feelings of anger, jealousy, meanness in outwardly slight situations known to oneself only
Emphasis on decision-making; any decision is better than none	Ability to live with some indecisiveness (multiple possibilities) even though it means living with some anxiety
Feeling of guilt toward someone who has denounced one for adequate or inadequate cause	Feeling of shame toward someone who trusts one if one is not meeting that trust
Emphasis on content of experience in work, leisure, personal relations	Emphasis on quality of experience, not only on content
Surmounting of guilt leads to righteousness	Transcending of shame may lead to sense of identity, freedom

This comparison, as well as Erikson's analysis of stages of development, would seem to suggest again that a sense of identity cannot be reached along the guilt axis alone, that more is needed than discarding specific wrong acts and substituting specific right acts for them. Can confronting experiences of shame full in the face be one clue to the discovery of what this something more is?

We cannot know, but it is interesting to speculate on what Emily Dickinson meant when she wrote:

> Shame need not crouch
> In such an earth as ours;
> Shame, stand erect,
> The universe is yours!

Clues to Identity

What follows is an attempt to suggest more concretely some attitudes and ways of life that may lead toward a sense of identity. Much of what is said here has been implied in what has gone before.

IDENTIFICATIONS AND IDENTITY

The combination of inner and outer direction inhering in a sense of identity suggests that developing a sense of identity includes both discovery of the kinds of identifications one may have with the life-style of one's own society and culture, or with wider groups and values, and an idiom of one's own that comprises but is distinct from these identifications. A sense of identity would seem—at least for some people—to demand bringing unconscious identifications into conscious awareness, becoming aware of the aspects of prescribed social roles with which they do and do not identify, entering into an engagement—positive or negative—with the society in which they live.

Some kind of answer to the question Where do I belong? is necessary for an answer to the question Who am I?

Virginia Woolf has described the predicament of finding oneself in a situation cut off from identifications. During the Second World War she wrote:

> I'm loosely anchored. Further, the war—our waiting while the knives sharpen for the operation—has taken away the outer wall of

security. No echo comes back. I have no surroundings. . . . Those familiar circumvolutions—those standards—which have for so many years given back an echo and so thickened my identity are all wide and wild as the desert now.[a]

The discovery of our place in our own society requires—at least for some individuals—seeing this society in the perspective of other societies and of history. It further requires some working hypothesis as to whether the limitations that this society and any other known society impose on human desires are an unchangeable "reality" inseparable from man's tragic fate, or a part of human history that can to some extent be changed by men. If a society that gives greater encouragement to varied human desires is conceived as a genuine possibility, then the questions of where our own social group and where we as a part of it stand in relation to such an enabling society become active questions.

From Hobbes to Freud runs an insistence on the inevitably confining nature of human society and on the inescapable and unending conflict between individual desires and the restrictions imposed by any social group in any conceivable historical situation. The influence of Darwin, however far this may have been from his intention, strengthened the idea of each against all. Nietzsche saw not only nineteenth-century, bourgeois, Christian society, but any society, as the enemy of individual man. Many contemporaries protest against being "members" of society; they think of themselves as entities over against the entity of society with the relation between the two hostile. Many happenings of the last twenty-five or fifty years have intensified the view that society is the enemy of the individual. Some forms of contemporary collectivism stress the *losing* of individual identity in the social group.

Is it possible for a person to find identifications with social groups in ways that mean not a losing but a finding of himself?

Rousseau and Hegel and Marx and some social scientists, such as Charles Horton Cooley, may have developed too easy verbal and abstract solutions to the question of how individual desires and group welfare can enhance each other. But many contemporary theorists do not even confront the problem or, if they do, regard it as beyond solution.

At least minimal adjustment of one's own wishes to whatever society one lives in is necessary for survival. But beyond this minimal adjustment, society is still viewed by many individuals and by many theories as something inherently alien to personal desires, something with which the individual must painfully "cope" and to which, at the expense of his own wishes, he must adapt.

Some psychologists and social scientists recognize different degrees and kinds of conflict between what may be regarded as biological and psychological impulses common to all men and the demands of society. But they draw different conclusions about these different degrees of disparity. For some it means only that the greater the gap between individual wishes and social demands the harder is the task of society to mold the individual to its design.[a]

Psychologists and psychoanalysts, if not social scientists, have given more encouragement to the adjustment of individuals to the realities of a given society than to personal differentiation and deviation from them. They frequently fail to give explicit recognition to the distinction between normal or healthy in terms of whatever are the generally accepted norms of the society and in terms of what is humanly desirable. If the psychoanalyst or the social scientist does not rigorously examine his own values in relation to those of society, he almost inevitably tends to accept tacitly the dominant values of the society as the norm of behavior, and to measure mental health and illness by these. Scientific objectivity, then, becomes indistinguishable from acceptance of social determinants. If human personality is thought to be understandable without reference to a specific social and historical situation, then this social "reality" does not need special analysis.[b]

Such social acquiescence or, if not acquiescence, reluctance to face directly the risks involved in any fundamental change in the social order appears even among those psychiatrists who are most aware of the restrictions our present society imposes on the development of human possibilities. Harry Stack Sullivan, for example, believed that in our time many personal psychological difficulties have their source, not in individual, but in social, pathology. Further, he believed that social pathologies are cumulative, so that "increasing uncertainty, insecurity, and discouragement" are "coming to be the common lot," [a] and that this degree of insecurity is a specific historical condition, not one rooted in the nature of man or of society. But he drew back from what might seem to be the next step in this chain of reasoning—that men should endeavor to bring about whatever fundamental institutional changes may be necessary to make society more favorable for human development. Instead he was reluctant to contemplate as much change and rebuilding in society as he thought necessary in individuals; and in dealing with social issues he suggested relying on a "traditional, almost accidental way of progress," [b] although he would certainly have thought tradition and accident an inadequate basis for the treatment of individuals. Although he undoubtedly recognized that in therapy it may be necessary for an individual to go through a period of chaos in order to reach a new stage of development, he did not recognize the possibility of a similar necessity in historical development. He condemned the person who is "sufficiently disturbed in his interpersonal relations to yearn for" a radical solution on the far side of chaos.[c] The cumulative effect of such thinking is a drawing away from the possibility of radical social change. Just because a psychiatrist like Sullivan recognized the importance of the social situation, this attitude may have more reactionary influence than that of a psychologist or pyschiatrist whose interest does not extend beyond the individual.

Erikson, even with all his insistence on the importance for the individual of identifications with the life-style of his culture, sees, at least to some extent, the difficulties this presents in the contemporary world. He speaks of the loss of identity among discharged veterans as a result of radical historical change, and says that the contemporary psychoanalyst who concentrates on the problems of the individual because it is easier than confronting the "infinitely more disquieting awareness" of the part that historical changes have played in creating these difficulties is helping to deflect energy from the collective tasks that must be faced.[a] This statement coming from a psychoanalyst is of great importance.

Another interpretation of the gap between individual desires and social demands is that the healthy personality is almost impossible of attainment in a society like our own, and, moreover, that in every known society the possibilities for full realization of individual capacities have always been restricted to a small part of the population. Here we sometimes find the reverse of the kind of reliance on tradition and accident for desired social change just described. Some social scientists who consider no study and planning too searching to apply to institutional change are content to rely on tradition and accident for the understanding of the individuals who compose society. They tend to regard careful investigation of what takes place within the individual personality as unnecessary and irrelevant "psychologizing" that encourages complacency about social issues and diverts attention from the necessities of social change.*

Marcuse, as noted above,† believes that psychologists and psychoanalysts who stress the possibilities of creative living in our present society are glossing over the coercive character of this society and are supporting reaction; and that Freud, with his insistence on the inherent hostility between individual desires and social demands, is the more radical social critic because he correctly describes the alienation of the individual in capitalist society.[b] Marcuse's translation of Freudian psychological determinism into Marxian historical determinism in order to demonstrate the repressions that capitalist society exerts on individual capacities is a sleight of hand that distorts Freud; but his treatment of Freud does not detract from the importance of his bringing into the open the extent to which this society does repress human capacities.

Any polarizing of psychology and history cripples the investigation of the issues that both psychologists and social scientists are trying to understand.

Here then is the problem. The evidence seems to show that

* Cf. pp. 107-17.

† Pp. 101, 117, 153 n.[1]

it is almost impossible for an individual to develop a sure sense of himself unless he can find aspects of his social situation with which he can clearly identify. For some persons identifications with family, neighborhood, or immediate community are apparently adequate. For others identifications with a larger community, such as the nation, are essential. Clear identifications are difficult when a country that describes itself as a nation of democracy, freedom, and peace practices ruthlessness toward less powerful peoples, support of fascism to fight Communism, and atomic warfare. The President of this humanitarian, Christian country has said of the atomic destruction of other peoples, ". . . the use of the atomic bomb would be on this basis . . . Does it advantage me or does it not when I get into a war? . . . If I thought the net was on my side I would use it instantly." [a]

Experiences of shame were described as sudden awareness of incongruity between oneself and the social situation, of exposure, in which an unexpected light is thrown on who one is. But this is a time that sharpens awareness that it is one's society, as well as oneself, that stands uncovered. Values, ways of life that one has accepted without question may appear in this new light to be cruel, hypocritical, destructive of the individual freedoms and possibilities they proclaim. If this is my society, my country, then the world is not good, I do not belong here, I want none of it—this, as well as self-insight may be the revelation of shame. Just as shame for one's parents and shame for others may be an even more searing experience than shame for oneself, so the questioning of certain dominant values presented by society can for some people be more disquieting than the questioning of one's own adequacy in living up to these values.

A special problem in cultural identifications is presented for parents and teachers who are critical of policies of their nation or of central characteristics of their immediate society. Many observers have pointed out that, as in situations of bombing during the war, children can endure a great amount of frustration, dislocation, and physical danger if they can go through these situations with the conviction that the adults who are involved in the situations know what they themselves are about and have assurance about the significance of what they are doing. But this does not altogether meet the hazards for the child who has difficulty in finding group identifications because the ideas of his parents place them and him in a minority group actively opposed to dominant policies.

David Garnett comments that, although he has come to believe that his parents and their closest friends were right in their opposition to the Boer War (in which there were British concentration camps where Boer women and children were allowed to die by hundreds in order to prevent them from cultivating the farms while their men were fighting), he, nevertheless, suffered permanent damage, not so much from being stoned by his schoolmates for being pro-Boer, as from not being able to identify as a British boy with the British cause.[a]

But what should his parents have done? He does not, and perhaps cannot, say. If his parents had been genuinely pro-British he might have come later to feel that they had influenced him to be parochial, cruel, and insensitive. If they had attempted to conceal from him their opposition to British policy he might have been unfortunately affected by, or have come to resent, their hypocrisy.[b] Could they have helped him toward identifications with a wider than national group that would have provided a sustaining equivalent of more immediate identifications?* Or can parents respect and enjoy the child's world more than they do and refrain from introducing adult concerns for which the child is not ready? In Garnett's situation this would have been impossible since he would have heard talk of the Boer War at school if not at home. One may be inclined to feel that an answer to this perplexity lies in the direction of less intrusion of parental values into the child's world, but this may run counter to what is also desirable—and neglected in our urban middle-class society—having a child

* There is also the question as to whether, if they had been able to provide these wider identifications, it could have been done without giving him at the same time a sense of moral superiority—of being in a special group—which has its own hazards.

be, according to his maturing capacities, a functioning part of the life of the social group.*

In finding conscious identifications with and beyond our own time and society, much turns upon the way we conceive realism, what meaning we give to "facing reality." Continually we are urged by therapists, by realists in foreign policy, by practical persons of various kinds to abandon sentimental dreams, idealistic utopias, and romanticism, and to face reality. Reality when so used almost always means limitation. The reality we should face is the limitations in ourselves, in other people, in the possibilities of human society. Rarely are we urged to face the reality of the slanting light of early morning and late afternoon, of Berlioz' "Luceat!," of Braque's colors, of human courage and integrity under stress, of delight in wit and laughter, of a child's expectancy, of the revelation of new human experience in unimagined openness and communication with another person, of the ranges of the possible.

Statements of realism, or of the reality principle, as acknowledgment of limitation, of adjusting to the *is* rather than dreaming of the *possible,* are well known. All of them are some version of Machiavelli's central tenet:

> . . . how one lives is so far distant from how one ought to live that he who neglects what is done for what ought to be done sooner effects his ruin than his preservation.

Edmund, as he ordered the death of Lear and Cordelia, followed the implications of this admonition for realistic identification with one's place and time in history:

> . . . men
> Are as the time is. To be tender-minded
> Does not become a sword.[a]

He continued his mandate to the Captain:

> Thy great employment
> Will not bear question.[b]

* See pp. 233-4 for further discussion of what is involved in the wider identifications of children.

And he said of himself:

> . . . for my state
> Stands on me to defend, not to debate.[a]

The difficulty with the realism of Machiavelli or of Edmund as a basis for finding social identifications is not that it focuses on what the time is but that it unduly restricts that focus. Interpretations of the human lot that stress only its limitations do not distinguish between natural limitations that are unalterable and social and historical limitations that can to some extent be changed by men.[b] They also omit reference to certain other phenomena as indubitable as tragedy. It is not necessary to be blind to the tragic limitations of human life to affirm the importance of as yet unrealized possibilities. History has been described by Joachim Schumacher as the attempt of man to make a home for himself in the world. This attempt need not be abandoned because there are limits beyond which it cannot go. Possibilities within these limits exceed anything thus far explored or imagined.

All realism and all identifications must be selective. No person and no society can grasp the whole of any historical situation. The most conforming person in the most monolithic society does not automatically take over identifications and combine them to form his own identity.[c]

But much tends at present to narrow our basis of choice. This constriction may be an interpretation of reality phrased in terms of deprivation, indulgence, or indifference in personal relations, of power and submission, reward and punishment, some form of psychological and moral scarcity. Or it may be phrased in the existentialist terms of death, inevitable human tragedy, and isolation. Or in the terms of an easy optimism of right and wrong choices. Any of these tends to emphasize what cannot be done. And this narrowed focus—applied to human nature, to the external world, to the understanding of other peoples and our own, to diplomatic options, to social roles in the United States—constantly intensifies itself. Each successive step in seeking an immediate reward, in meeting what is regarded as an immediate threat, in concentrating on the most obviously coercive next steps, involves a more constricted focus and further distortion of perspective, and makes the subsequent steps seem inevitable, allowing still less choice.

Realism that excludes the longer, enduring purposes of men and men's unrealized dreams is less than full realism.[a] Dreams need not be illusions. We can constantly attempt to distinguish between futile utopianism and the possibilities of the future implicit in the present. Insistence on what are called realistic limits has always meant that they are assumed to be narrower and more rigid than they potentially are. History may be viewed as a process of pushing back walls of inevitability, of turning what have been thought to be inescapable limitations into human possibilities. The utopianism of one era has repeatedly become the basic norm of decency for the next. Some of the developments that make discovery of identity more difficult at present—the simultaneous impact of different cultures and perspectives, the exposure to world-wide instead of to more localized events—also extend the range of selectivity. Instead of lamenting, as a threat, the distintegration of many traditional values and the lack of clear definition with which our historical period presents us, we may attempt to understand and to use the very conflicts and ambiguities of the time to open the way for realization of new possibilities.

ENGAGEMENT WITH CONTEMPORARY CONFLICTS

If we are to be participants in our particular phase of history, we cannot remain unaware of the dimensions of contemporary conflicts. Paradoxically, I believe that we could live less painfully with the almost overwhelming conflicts of the present, and find more of ourselves in the midst of them, if instead of protecting ourselves from them, we allowed ourselves to realize more fully their immense difficulty. Such awareness requires more than seeking here-and-now right answers to the questions these conflicts embody: Is the man innocent or guilty? Does he put love of country before other loyalties or is he a traitor without integrity? Is he good and wise or evil and foolish? Is a particular people peaceful or imperialistic? Which are the freedom-loving and which are the totalitarian nations? What action will "solve" a particular problem? We have little realization of the historical period we are living in if we think that its central issues can be stated in such terms.

Sir Laurence Olivier's version of *Hamlet* illustrates the wiping out of conflicts by oversimplification. The subtitle of the film, "The tragedy of a man who could not make up his mind," implies that if Hamlet had only been a more decisive character all would have been well. Such a conception ignores the fact that the questions Hamlet struggled with were real questions: Was the ghost a devil or was it his father? Was Claudius, was Gertrude, guilty of murder? Of adultery? If guilty, was justice best served by a life for a life? What does violent action solve? What is life after death? If he killed Claudius at prayer would he be rewarding, not punishing, him? Must one renounce love as weakness or diversion if one is committed to a cause? Conflicts between past traditions and looking to the future, between different religious views of the world, different theories of spirits, different historical forms of reality, all entered in. Decisive action could not take the place of human and historical understanding.

Our age also presents issues of belief, of moral judgment, of loyalties, of personal responsibility, of historical change that do not allow obvious right answers that can resolve the conflict, dispose of the issue, give the satisfaction of "making up one's mind," and escaping from quandary into action.

Racial discrimination, says the World Council of Churches, is not only "an unutterable offense against God" but where it is the law Christians may properly "feel bound to disobey such law." [a] In 1956 and 1957 the Koinonia Community in Georgia, a nondenominational Christian agricultural community, was subjected to shooting, bombing, and other forms of violence because they practiced Christian fellowship in maintaining an interracial community. Similar incidents of violence have occurred in putting desegregation into effect in other parts of the United States. In such situations as these, or of the refusal of a group of German physicists to work on the atomic bomb or of conscientious objectors to engage in military service, how does one reconcile loyalty to one's immediate community or to one's country with loyalty to one's conscience and to humanity?

The difficulties of accepting reality and achieving decisiveness in such situations is recognized by some psychoanalysts. Meerloo, for example, describes the choice that many witnesses before Congressional committees have to make between contempt of Congress and contempt of human relations.

> Administrators may conceivably discover a few alleged "traitors" by compelling witnesses to betray their former friends, but at the same time they compel people to betray friendships.
>
> . . . By forcing a man to betray his inner feelings and himself, we actually make it easier for him to betray the larger community at some future date.[a]

Are such protests an appeal from the sovereignty of one's own society to the "sovereignty of mankind"? In such situations do we encounter again the question: If one may feel guilt for disobedience to a particular law are there basic human decencies that one cannot violate without shame?

Some analyses by R. H. S. Crossman are exceptional in their grasp of the nature and scope of the conflicts—in an age of total warfare, colonial revolution, racial desegregation, and national and international organization—between submission to authority and reliance on one's own moral judgment, between loyalty to one's society or country and loyalty to one's conscience or to humanity. Writing of Alan Moorehead's *The Traitors: The Double Life of Fuchs, Pontecorvo and Nunn May,*[b] Crossman says:

> . . . there is one resemblance between the 1550's and the 1950's. The Elizabethans, like ourselves, lived in an Age of Treason. Then, too, an honourable man could be faced with the choice of betraying his country or his creed. . . . To the Victorian, treason was quite simply a monstrous crime; to the Elizabethans, it was the central problem of politics. Whether a political conspiracy is justified; how to conspire nobly; how to face death if the conspiracy fails; these are the questions which tormented the characters in Shakespeare's plays. . . . To assume that any traitor must be a villain is to make nonsense of *Julius Caesar* and most of the Histories.

Frequently, in order to preserve society against the State, men have been forced to break their solemn oaths.

Paradoxically, Mr. Moorehead has selected for condemnation the flaw in Fuchs' Communism which ultimately brought him to volunteer [his] confession. . . . The son of a Lutheran pastor, he retained the Protestant conscience. Without a minority of men and women who are willing to be "martyrs to their conscience," representative government must lapse into corruption. This belief in the inner light is, of course, condemned, by Communists as well as Catholics, as spiritual arrogance. . . . The political non-conformists, who are the leaven of democracy, cannot accept this ethic. With John Locke they claim the right of revolution against established authority, whether it is a Bishop, a Party Executive, or the State itself.[a]

Crossman compares "the millennialism, the iconoclasm, and the sense of predestined victory, which inspired and often perverted the Protestant struggle for religious and national independence" with the hopes "which now impel the millions of Asia and Africa to accept Communist absolutism."[b]

. . . Englishmen . . . realize that the victories of the great heresy spring from the corruption of our own orthodoxy. . . . Once again the propagation of the Faith has become entangled with the propaganda of the Prince. . . . Since war—fought ostensibly for the highest principle—is the normal state of the new Elizabethan man, patriotism demands the unqualified acceptance of the established ideology. But the link between patriotism and personal conscience may at any moment be broken by a shift of alliances which transforms a servant of Lucifer into a servant of God.[c]

The traitors, says the *Economist,* were guilty of the "sin of pride." Pride is regarded as a sin when it is treachery to the established government, as a virtue, especially in retrospect, when it is "independence of conscience." But the *Economist* is not unaware of the uneasy relation between the Faith and the Prince—"when Fuchs came to England, Germany was the enemy and Russia the ally."[d] Freud recognized this conflict between the Faith and the Prince in the First World War. "The individual citizen can prove with dismay in this war . . . that the state forbids him to do wrong not because it wishes to do away with wrong doing but because it wishes to monopolize it, like salt and tobacco." [a]

Morton Grodzins delineates in more detail the complexity in a time of social upheaval of the choice between patriotism to one's country and "above all nations humanity." [b] To the Japanese-American citizens who were forcibly evacuated to "relocation centers" during the Second World War the issue frequently presented itself as a conflict between loyalty to their belief in democracy and to their belief in the United States.

The 8 to 52 per cent of the Japanese-American citizens interned in the camps who refused to take a loyalty oath to the United States*—more than six thousand American citizens—were, according to Grodzins, not loyal for the following reasons: They did not want to support by a declaration of loyalty what they believed to be unjust persecution, discrimination, and second-class citizenship; they did not want to betray or to be disloyal to their families; they did not want again to undergo forcible removal—this time from the camps—with the risk that they could not survive economically; some preferred, or had come to prefer, the Japanese way of life.[c]

From the evidence of the Japanese-Americans who refused to take a loyalty oath to the United States, as well as from other examples of disloyalty (or treachery), Grodzins concludes that a disloyal person, including the most clearly marked traitor, is in his own eyes not disloyal but loyal to something other and more worthy of allegiance, some larger ideal.[d] Sir Thomas More, condemned for refusing to swear to the supremacy of a Protestant king, went to his death with the words, "I die the King's good servant, but God's first." [e] Grodzins makes the important point that if all ideas and ideals could be explained—or explained away—in terms of the personal or economic and social factors that gave rise to them there would be no way of explaining the independent thrust they exhibit. "The honorable may betray virtue, king, country, or home; but the honorable do not betray their conception of honor. Those who put

* The percentages varied according to the kind of treatment the Japanese-Americans had received in the different camps. At the camp where the largest per cent refused to take the loyalty oath conditions were particularly bad.

first things first may head their list with mankind, world government, salvation. If these come into conflict with nation, nation is put second."[a] All patriots, therefore, are potential traitors if they are committed to other values even more important to them than their patriotism—artistic or scientific or religious truth, justice, or humanity.

None of these considerations minimizes the importance of identifications with one's country, but they point to the naïveté of taking loyalty to country as necessarily the basic or central loyalty, synonymous with integrity, and treachery as a priori the supreme crime, a total loss of integrity.[b] Such a conception dwarfs human nature and underestimates the ranges of honor and the complexities of history.

It is strange that as perceptive an observer as Meerloo in discussing treason ignores all questions of the sort raised by Crossman and Grodzins, all the social and historical factors that make loyalty to country and treason genuine issues, treats patriotism to the United States as an unquestionable central loyalty, and treason as purely a problem of individual pathology. He assumes that "the enemy" is wrong whoever the enemy is. He appears to recognize no independent validity in systems of ideas and ideals beyond loosely used "democratic" and "totalitarian." In his view the key to treason is "self-betrayal." "The germ of treason arises first in the individual's compromises with his own principles and beliefs. . . . It is because all of us do doubt ourselves . . . and because we may see in ourselves a potential traitor, that the word 'treason' has such highly emotional appeal."[c]

For citizens of other nations or of other times we recognize that the nation as an entity that demands loyalty may conflict with wider personal or social faiths that demand loyalty. For ourselves, we continually hope that personal integrity, political and religious belief, scientific and artistic honor, fidelity to family and friends, and patriotism to country can be woven together into one seamless whole. We resist recognition that there are times, and that our own is one of them, when this unity is difficult or impossible to achieve.

Thus we make heavy going of the conflicts presented to a

scientist in the position of Robert Oppenheimer for whom loyalty to family and friends, scientific honor, patriotism, and human decency are actually in conflict. These are not issues between morality and immorality but among conflicting moralities. A scientific discoverer or any other discoverer is inevitably a questioner. Security regulations in contemporary America discourage questioning and insist that "a man abandon interior quarrel when he assumes a public responsibility." [a] Such escape from moral responsibility as a requirement for public service contributes neither to the security of the country nor to the identity or integrity of the individual.

Oversimplification of conflicts in fundamental moralities frequently leads us in America to underestimate a situation that has been of concern to recent French writers: the act of courage, seemingly useless, that one may nevertheless require of oneself. In its assertion of human values and human dignity beyond those of any particular social code, such an act of courage is the counterpart of shame. It demands action that has no discernible pragmatic outcome but is an affirmation of belief in oneself and of meaning in the world. The choice between doing and not doing an act that may effect nothing but is nevertheless crucial for maintaining the sense of one's own humanity presented itself continuously to the persons Camus describes in *The Plague*. It is the theme of Bloch-Michel's *The Witness,* in which the central character could not in the end forgive himself for not sharing the apparently useless heroism of his wife, who took part in the Resistance because she could not withhold herself from life.[b] The same affirmation of significance beyond the immediate appears in the action of the Polish Jews who sang as they went into the gas chambers.

Similar problems presented themselves to Rubashev in *Darkness at Noon* and to the characters in *The Case of Comrade Tulayev.*[c] The importance of such studies is missed if they are regarded as political tracts for one side or the other. They show the genuine conflicts among different moralities for individuals who have become disillusioned with beliefs to which they were committed and for which they had fought, but who cannot bring themselves to betray a cause that may still hold some promise for the future. An analysis in terms of guilt and right-doing does not cover such situations any more than it explains traitors in a period of social upheaval, although guilt certainly enters into these conflicts. The difficulties lie not in the violation of a particular code, but in conflicts between codes, each compelling loyalty.

Entering fully into the nature of contemporary conflicts calls upon one to make choices beyond coping with difficulties to gain security; beyond the polarity of good on the one side, evil on the other; in terms of multiple possibilities. As Goldstein has shown, the sick person cannot live in terms of possibilities; he must have a decisive, unambiguous, conflict-free situation in order to exist at all.* Acting in the faith that there may be ranges of individual and social development as yet unknown requires ability to live with ambiguity and varied probabilities and possibilities.[a] Such a view enlarges the concept of morality. Morality becomes, in Guyau's words, not "I must, therefore I can," but "I can, therefore I must"; "To feel inwardly the greatest that one is capable of doing is really the first consciousness of what it is one's duty to do." [b] It is acting in good faith. It calls for an entirely different measure of moral strength, a measurement of oneself and of one's society against both a larger historical and a larger human perspective.

IDENTIFICATIONS BEYOND PRESCRIBED ROLES

The idea of entering fully into the conflicts of our historical period and living in terms of a wider range of possibilities in oneself and in one's society raises again the question of what more than the combination of prescribed social roles enables an individual to say: This is I.

Three further questions arise here:

What are the processes by which certain aspects of identifications with parents and with cultural roles are accepted and others rejected, and by which those accepted are woven into a new *Gestalt*?

* See pp. 144-5.

What enables some individuals more than others to endure frustration, to forego identifications with their immediate society, and to find identifications with wider, longer-range, and more diversified human values?

Are there identifications that derive less from the particular features of the society in which an individual has been bred than from characteristics and aspirations both more particular to individuals and more common to humanity? *

Attempts to answer these questions go into largely undiscovered country. Recent social theory, particularly the work of Durkheim, Parsons, and Merton, has taken note of deviance and *anomie*. But it remains true that in psychology and in social science in general more attention is still given to adaptation and adjustment to approved social roles and values than to deviation from them. And deviance is far too readily codified in oversimplified terms of genius or of rebellion or, even, of individual pathology.

All that has been said about shame as a revealing of one's society as well as of oneself points beyond complete cultural relativism toward the possibility of more universal human values. There seem to be indications of aspirations of the self that go beyond the demands of society, requirements of oneself that exceed social demands, perspectives against which one places the demands of one's own society.

In one form or another, the question of how one forms one's own idiom has been recurrent throughout our history. How do we explain Amos, Socrates, Tycho Brahe, Galileo, Martin Luther, Freud, Cézanne, Rilke, Stephen Hero, Black Boy—or prophets, rebels, artists, or other innovators whose names are unknown—whose sense of self is related to ideals that they conceive as widely human and at the same time peculiarly their own?

Heraclitus asserted man's moral autonomy in opposition to religious belief in a tutelary spirit; he distinguished life as individuated in men from other life processes by its capacity for

* Cf. the various places where this question has been raised earlier, pp. 22, 35-7.

heightening its own status. This heightening of oneself beyond cultural demands is precisely what is involved in discovery of identity.

In Aristotle's view the life of each individual was governed by a law of its own through the unfolding of which each person attained his own separate individuality, his own "true" nature. This conception of development influenced such a very different person as St. Augustine and, in more recent times, Ortega y Gasset.

Keats sought to account for the varieties of differentiation from the culture in terms somewhat closer to our own:

> Man is originally 'a poor forked creature' . . . subject to the same mischances as the beasts of the forest. . . . Call the world . . . 'The vale of soul-making.' . . . There may be intelligence or sparks of the divinity in millions—but they are not souls until they acquire identity, till each one is personally itself. . . . I will call the *world* a School instituted for the purpose of teaching little children to read—I will call the *human heart* the *horn Book* read in that School—and I will call the *Child able to read, the Soul* made from that *School* and its *hornbook*. . . . Not merely is the Heart a Hornbook, It is the Minds Bible, it is the Minds experience, it is the text from which the mind or intelligence sucks its identity. As various as the Lives of Men are—so various become their Souls . . . what are the provings of [man's] heart but fortifiers and alterers of his nature? and what is his altered nature but his soul?—and what was his Soul before it came into the world and had these provings and alterations and perfectionings?—An intelligence—without Identity—and how is this Identity to be made? Through the medium of the Heart? and how is the Heart to become this Medium but in a world of Circumstances? [a]

Some men and women as they grow older become less differentiated from, more and more replicas of, or masks formed by, their society. This can be seen from their successive portraits and from their literary and artistic work. Advancing years mean to them more need of the protection of being like others, less of the risk involved in the search for their own way of life. Others develop with added years more sureness and deeprootedness in themselves in relation to the world. Their faces, their letters, and their published writings or artistic productions become more forthright, more genuinely individual as they grow older. This was true of Goethe, of T. H. Huxley, of Yeats, of Einstein.

The larger-than-immediate roles and values with which one can identify include the nonpersonal as well as the personal world. Work, relationship to, and discovery in, the nonpersonal world is not only or always a compensation or substitute for frustrated personal or sexual impulses. As the child begins to distinguish himself from the world around him and to acquire a growing sense of himself and of his own desires, this sense of self grows step by step with interest in the reality of the external world. The discovery of what is reality in nonpersonal things in themselves not related to one's personality is an indispensable part of discovering what is one's personality.

Piaget has described the child's early lack of distinction between inner and outer, subject and object, psychological and physical, living and nonliving. Schilder and Schachtel have amplified the account of the slow development of the sense of self as something different from the world of other people and of things, as this outer world at the same time becomes recognizable as something different from oneself.

Schachtel speaks of the importance of "the variety of the playful approach, as contrasted with the narrow directedness of the need-driven approach" in developing a child's sense of the world of social demands and of objects and of himself as related to, but distinct from, both.[a]

Curiosity, the desire for knowledge, the wish to orient oneself in the world one lives in—and finally the posing of man's eternal questions, "Who am I?" "What is this world around me?" "What can I hope for?" "What should I do?"—all these do not develop under the pressure of relentless need or of fear for one's life. They develop when man can pause to think, when the child is free to wonder and to explore. . . . They represent man's distinctive capacity to develop *interest*—the autonomous interest which alone permits the full encounter with the object.[b]

The child's reflective focussing on his own feelings and experiences constitutes the last step in the development of focal attention, and accompanies the development of the idea of "I" and the autobiographical memory—that is, the concept of the continuity of the self.[a]

In the discovery and creation of oneself in relation to and differentiated from social codes, both one's self-image, the picture of what one is, and one's self-ideal, the picture of what one would like to be, are involved. Different degrees and kinds of congruence between the two and between both and the life-style approved by the culture emerge in the process of developing identity.

As noted above,* there is much confusion about these terms, about the parts of the self they denote, and the ways in which these parts function in the developing personality. The superego of Freud is relatively clear. It is a prohibiting, restraining, guilt-producing part of the self compounded from instinctual drives, desire for parental approval, and parental threats and prohibitions which have become internalized through identification with the parents or with the parents' ideals. The self-ideal in Piers' sense is concerned, not with violation of taboos, but with long-term purposes and goals.[b]

There is need to explore further, not only the sources of the idea of self and of the self-ideal, but also the kinds of relations there may be between them. One basis for distinction between different kinds of relations between the self and the self-ideal is the difference between a sense of identity formed primarily on what I have called the guilt axis (in Piers' words, formed in terms of the prohibiting superego) and a sense of identity formed primarily on what I have called the shame axis (in Piers' words, formed in terms of the ego-ideal). Individuals tend to find continuity in their lives either by means of basic emphasis on what others have taught them they should do and —more especially—should not do, or by means of emphasis on discovering their own lines of direction. Learning to know oneself is in part the ability to distinguish between these two ways of growth. In our society a person is inclined to be more specifically conscious of behavior on the guilt axis, of transgres-

* Pp. 166-71.

sions that are culturally defined and redeemable, and of their counterparts that add up role by role to a righteous, mature, adjusted life. He can perhaps at relatively small emotional expense fulfill the requirements society makes of him. But identity built on the guilt axis may be less enduring, more likely to break down into its parts. If its loyalties are based mainly on social requirements, the sense of self may change if these requirements shift.

Identity based more on the shame axis may go deeper and be more of a continuous process of creation with less easily dissipated *Gestalts*. Shame, while touched off by a specific, often outwardly trivial, occurrence initially felt as revealing one's own inadequacies, may also confront one with unrecognized desires of one's own and the inadequacy of society in giving expression to these desires. There is a natural tendency to seek cover from such experiences since the culture has little place for revelations of the inmost self or of the central dynamics of the society. But it is the whole purpose of oneself and of one's society that invites re-examination in the light of these experiences. Selective fulfilling of social roles when it occurs then becomes part of a continuing process rather than a series of isolable acts Stubborn and minute control is replaced by the unfolding of the spirit. In a society more directly and variously expressive of human desires the guilt axis and the shame axis, role fulfillment and personal fulfillment, might more nearly coincide.

Although in many experiences both guilt and shame are involved, at times the differences between adaptation to the social roles demanded by society and the demands of one's own life appear in sharp contrast. Of Aleksei Aleksandrovitch, Tolstoy says:

> [He] was now standing face to face with life, with the possibility that his wife was in love with someone else . . . and this seemed to him very senseless and incomprehensible, because it was life itself. All his life he had lived and labored in a round of official duties concerned with the reflections of life. And whenever he came in contact with life itself he was revolted by it. Now he experienced a sensation such as a man feels, who, passing calmly over a bridge

above a precipice, suddenly discovers that the arch is broken, and that the abyss yawns beneath his feet.

This abyss was actual life; the bridge—the artificial life he had been living.[a]

Confronting, instead of quickly covering, an experience of shame as revelation of oneself and of society—facing "actual life"—requires an ability to risk, if necessary to endure, disappointment, frustration, and ridicule. Commitment to any position or to any loyalty, like commitment to another person, involves the risk of being wrong and the risk of being ridiculous. It is *relatively* easy to take even difficult action if one is sure that one is right, that one has grasped the truth of a situation; it is relatively easy to entertain multiple possibilities of truth and of right action if one remains a spectator on the sidelines. Far more difficult than either is to give everything one is in supporting all the truth that one can see at any given time, with full awareness that there are other possibilities and that further knowledge may enlarge and revise the hypotheses on which one has risked everything. Engagement with life and with history—self-discovery and further discovery of the world—has always involved just such risks.

There is no easy way to distinguish between elements of dissolution and of promise in an era of the destruction of an old order and the birth of a new, between chaos that is only destructive and chaos that heralds the future, or even between that which is appropriately called order and that which is called disorder. Many people thought that they were living in a society of order and secure values in England at a time when children were working twelve hours a day in the mines and the mills.

But the culture within which one may discover identifications is more than a geographical unit, more than a national concept, more than a particular historical period. History is more than the present, more than aspects of the past now dominant; it has other available traditions and various possible futures. The values associated with the importance of individual idiom, with human relations, freedom, and democracy, which we cherish as our cultural identifications, may be found in new forms in other parts of the world. We may extend the range of selectivity that inheres in any social situation to include wider areas, longer historical perspectives, closer examination of varied possibilities and of actual options within the present.

Harder than our own difficulties in living in such wider perspectives is contemplating such difficulties for the next generation. We would have them encounter what the world can be at the time they are living in it. But we shrink from what this encounter involves. We do not want their lives to be subject to the hazards of our own—or of their own—beliefs.

But we cannot have it this way. We want them to be intelligent and discerning. And we know that it is often the persons who have the greatest intelligence and awareness who are also most vulnerable to the inhumanities and hypocrisies of society and the least ready to make the compromises necessary for adjustment. They have a selectivity that does not allow them to accept passively.* How do we meet the perplexities of our children? How do we respond to the questions of our students about what it is to be mature, how one decides when to stand fast to a loyalty, when to modify and to conform[a]—all their contemporary versions of Kant's three questions: How can I know? What can I hope? What should I do? How and when do we prepare our children and our students for transition from the kind of personal responsiveness and support for their expectations that home and college may offer to a more impersonal and contradictory world? And how help them to discover wider identifications through which they can find continuities?

* Erikson says of Darwin, "I do not wish to speculate here on the dynamics of a psychoneurosis in a man like Darwin. But I do know that a peculiar malaise can befall those who have seen too much, who, in ascertaining new facts in a spirit seemingly as innocent as that of a child who builds with blocks, begin to perceive of the place of these facts in the moral climate of their day . . . a creative man has no choice. He may come across his supreme task almost accidentally. But once the issue is joined, his task proves to be at the same time intimately related to his most personal conflicts, to his superior selective perception, and to the stubbornness of his one-way will: he must . . . test . . . whether the established world will crush him, or whether he will disestablish a sector of this world's outworn fundaments and make place for a new one." ("The First Psychoanalyst," *The Yale Review*, Vol. XLVI, No. 1, Sept. 1956, pp. 42-3.)

If greater awareness may make them more unprotected against the impact of the contradictions in society it may also give them more sturdy capacity, in Heraclitus' words, to heighten their own stature and to discern and ally themselves with men and values over wider ranges of time and space. The sense of identity that may be the outcome of the confrontation of the implications of shame is a lifelong process of discovery. Nor is it an even or a continuous process of discovery.

This again is truer the more intelligent, the more responsive, and hence the more aware and vulnerable the person is. Freud speaks of the "repeated adolescence" of creative minds which he ascribes to himself as well as to his friend Fliess. Goethe believed that while most people are young only once, there are some—and these the most gifted—who experience their youth repeatedly.[a] Such individuals must recurrently face what those who adapt more easily to social requirements settle in late adolescence. "The 'normal' individual combines the various prohibitions and challenges of the ego-ideal in a sober, modest, and workable unit, well anchored in a set of techniques and in the roles that go with them. The restless individual must, for better or for worse . . . [continually reassert] his ego identity."[b]

Although the realization of identity is something more than and different from identification with parents and with social roles approved by society, the ways in which it is different from these identifications can be too simply conceived. Some restatements of the individual-group relation assume something like polar opposites between individuation and being a part of humanity.

Plato, Aristotle, and Kant believed that the most significant characteristic of men is their capacity for reason, and that affect, desire, and feeling are less important "accidental" features. They then drew the conclusion that only those aspects of human behavior that have to do with reason can be studied or are worth studying. Many philosophical, psychological, and social theories have been built on this assumption of the basic rationality of man. Freud in some sense reversed it, making emotion rather than reason basic in human beings, then attempting to classify emotions and to trace developmental stages that are alike, or differ only in quantitative distribution, for all men.

Like Freud, although with different wording and emphasis, Harry Stack Sullivan bases his theory and his therapy on the observation that we are all "more simply human" than we are healthy or diseased, normal or abnormal.[a] But Sullivan contrasts being more simply human with individual uniqueness.[a] Common humanity and individual uniqueness are not, I believe, Platonic opposites, as Sullivan suggests, but Hegelian opposites, in the sense that each is part of and necessary to the other.

An awareness of unique, precise detail as a universalizing as well as an individualizing experience appears in the great novelists and poets. The shape of Dmitri's toes, Dorothea's experience in Rome,[c] the particular quality of Flora's relation to her father,[d] were peculiar to them; no other human being ever had precisely these characteristics or experiences. The expression on the face of the little Princess, Prince Andrey's wife, in childbirth; the approaches and withdrawals in the conversations between Andrey and Pierre; Marya's blushes; the length of Natasha's skirt at her first ball; Natasha's changes of mood at the opera; Prince Andrey's feeling as he listened to Natasha sing; Petya's love of raisins—nothing could be more particular to the individuals involved, yet is it not just these things that make *War and Peace* universally human?

Every individual has some qualities and ways of experiencing that are his own, and it is this fact as well as things that can be called common, shared human characteristics that make him a member of humanity. It is in part the very uniqueness of every individual that makes him, not only a member of a family, race, nation, or class, but a human being.

RELATIONS WITH OTHER PERSONS

It is not necessary to go as far as Sullivan does, in saying that what one *is* is one's personal relations, to recognize the crucial importance in the search for identity of the way one views and engages with other individuals. Relations with other persons are something different from selective identifications with aspects of one's immediate social situation or with wider values. Both are involved, but neither comprehends all of person-to-person relations.

In personal relations, as in other phases of life, guilt-axis and shame-axis orientations are frequently interwoven in a particular experience. But to a person who lives and views experience primarily along the guilt-righteousness axis other persons tend to be primarily external and instrumental to himself or—another version of the same thing—he instrumental to them. This is true whether he regards them (or himself in relation to them) as indulgent or depriving agents administering pleasure or pain, as representing certain social roles, or as members of an audience who mete out approval or scorn. To a person oriented more to the shame-identity axis, other persons, the They, or at least some of them, are parts of himself as he is part of them.

The first tends to regard both others and himself as instruments, remaining external to each other. He must always weigh and appraise and be on guard against committing himself. From others, he should seek approval, indulgence, contributions to his pleasure. For others, he should do the right thing, meet the appropriate standards, fulfill the designated social roles. He should never lose sight of what they will think of what he does and how that will affect him. Appraisal tends to be always present. Trust is in abeyance.

In our society "emotional" is frequently used as a derogatory term. Developing emotional maturity is more often conceived in terms of training a child in what he should *not* feel and in controlling the expression of his feelings than in extending the range and depth of his emotions and their expression.*

A person who lives more on the shame-identity or shame-freedom axis, and who opens himself to his own emotions, faces other difficulties and other possibilities. There is not only more question of what I think of what I do and how it will affect

* Scheler points out that the term "sympathy" is often wrongly confined to pity or compassion. Sympathy with suffering (*Mitleid*) and sympathy with joy (*Mitfreude*) are two different things often confused, and the second is frequently neglected in the study of the first. (V. J. McGill, "Scheler's Theory of Sympathy and Love," "Symposium on the Philosophy of Max Scheler," *Philosophy and Phenomenological Research,* Vol. II, No. 3, Mar. 1952, p. 276.)

others. Much more important, there is more ability to see the world through the eyes of another person, with another instead of myself as the center. The "I" is both more separate from, and more related to, other persons.

The blunting of the discovery by individuals of their own identity and their use of other persons as instrumental objects was the basis of Marx's indictment of capitalist industrialism, which, with varying degrees of explicitness, Fromm, Erikson, Marcuse, as well as some social scientists, follow.

> Only in community with others has each individual the means of cultivating his gifts in all directions. . . . In the real community the individuals obtain their freedom in and through their association.
>
> Competition makes individuals, not only the bourgeois but still more the workers, mutually hostile, in spite of the fact that it brings them together.[a]

Marx believed that present society "generates those false selves which make of our lives comedies and tragedies of mistaken identity." In the situation Marx hoped for, "No longer is each individual haunted by an alien 'I' detached from his daily life . . . the drama of the socialist revolution—and its pathos—is a drama of self-creation. . . . Making oneself would seem to be a different process from recognizing oneself as an already existing, if hidden, 'I'."[b]

Much depends upon whether one believes that isolation and alienation are inevitable in man's fate or that openness of communication between persons, mutual discovery, and love are actual possibilities. But even if one faces in the direction of trust and the possibility of discovery, the development of relations of mutuality is not easy.

When Freud says that human relations almost always end in disappointment and a cutting down of hopes to meet reality,*

* Edith Weigert adds that repeated disappointment of expectation leads even to a denial of the expectations themselves. ("Existentialism and Its Relations to Psychotherapy," *Psychiatry*, Vol. 12, No. 4, Nov. 1949.) Meerloo believes that for many persons today fear of human relations is greater than fear of death; they are afraid to take the emotional responsibility of having an emotional involvement with their fellow beings. (*The Rape of the Mind*, World Publishing Co., 1956, pp. 163-4.)

he is describing what does happen in many, if not most, personal relations in our society. Rarely, perhaps, do the particular personal qualities of individuals that can bring the greatest mutual fulfillment coincide with the appropriate, socially approved roles. Certain parts of the personality often have to be submerged for the fulfillment of others. This is why, even in our society, which ostensibly gives great importance to love as the basis for marriage, counselors who give advice on marriage tend to warn against reliance on romantic love and to stress companionship, comparable background, and socially approved roles as a firmer foundation for marital happiness. This is already a denial in advance of certain possibilities.

It may be that in any known society mutuality and trust that make possible profound openness between persons, and the finding of oneself in and through others, are all but impossible. To some extent limitations of mutuality because of the nature of human beings and of circumstances, as well as loss through death, are part of the human lot. Just as in one lifetime only a limited range of a person's possible ways of expression may be fulfilled, so in any one relation it may be that only some ranges of mutual love that each person brings to it can be realized.

But with all the inevitable limitations, it is questionable whether loneliness and the substitution of roles for mutual openness need to characterize person-to-person relations as largely as they do at present. Questions about other possibilities cut to the roots of assumptions about human nature and personal relations. Assumptions about the outgrowth of intimacy and assumptions about the effect of the passage of time are separately involved but related. Time necessarily brings changes in any relation, and one must be prepared to recognize these changes and to grow and change with time. But if one can believe that it is possible for the greater knowledge that two persons may acquire of each other in the course of time to bring also greater respect and love, then—beyond the inevitabilities of human life cycles—one need not fear time. Can one have faith that with certain other persons greater openness can increase understanding, respect, and love? That with them increasing intimacy can be, not a corroding, but a deepening and enriching process?

E. M. Forster points out the contrast between Proust's lack of faith and Dante's faith in the possibilities in human intimacy.[a] Proust believed that the fonder we are of people the less we understand and respect them; Dante that the fonder we are of people the greater is our understanding. To Dante increased knowledge was love, love knowledge. For Proust, as for Freud, time eventually destroys love; for Dante expansion of time makes love more possible.* Love can become an intensification of seeing, a looking into hidden possibilities.

Recognizing the extent to which people do use other persons as objects for their own satisfaction and security, and to which greater intimacy and the passage of time do diminish love, we still find exceptions, and it is important to try to discover the nature of these exceptions and of the conditions that seem to permit or foster them.[b]

Enlarging the possibilities of mutual love depends upon risking exposure. This risk of exposure can come about only with respect for oneself, respect for the other person, and recognition of nonpersonal values and loyalties that both persons respect. Through such love one comes to know the meaning of exposure without shame, and of shame transformed by being understood and shared. Aristotle distinguishes between feeling ashamed of things shameful "according to common opinion" and things shameful "in very truth." [c] In love there can be the exploring together of the meaning of things shameful "in very truth."

* Sartre, like Freud and Proust, believes that intimacy and satisfaction of desire tends to diminish love and to diminish oneself: ". . . the amorous intuition is . . . an ideal out of reach. The more I am loved, the more I lose my *being*. . . . In the second place the Other's awakening is always possible; at any moment he can make me appear as an object—hence the lover's perpetual insecurity. In the third place love is an absolute which is perpetually *made relative* by others . . . pleasure is the death and the failure of desire. It is the death of desire because it is not only its fulfillment but its limit and its end . . . pleasure . . . is *attention to the incarnation of the For-itself which is reflected-on* and by the same token it is forgetful of the Other's incarnation. (*Being and Nothingness*, Philosophical Library, 1956, pp. 377, 397.)

Then shall the fall further the flight in me

In mutual trust and love there can be no incongruous or inappropriate words or behavior. Dropping the protection of role-playing, letting oneself go freely in risking incongruity and inappropriateness is one of the delights of trusted love. Exposure can be exposure of the diversity of the good, the hopeful, the tender, as well as of what may be in other circumstances accounted shameful.

Love casts out fear. Shakespeare shares this Biblical emphasis. Unlike Freud, he contrasts love, not with hate, but with fear. Love is strong and unshaken; fear is weak, palehearted, shuddering, trembling. Fear casts out love. Mutual love is incompatible with desire for power over other persons. Macbeth's retribution was the retreat of love before fear following desire for power.

> Those he commands move only in command,
> Nothing in love . . .[a]

> . . . I am cabin'd, cribb'd, confin'd, bound in
> To saucy doubts and fears.[b]

Richard II saw that

> The love of wicked men converts to fear,
> That fear to hate . . .[c]

For Donne love encompasses fear as well as space and time.

> And now good-morrow to our waking souls,
> Which watch not one another out of fear;
> For love all love of other sights controls,
> And makes one little room an every where.

The experience of deep engagement with and commitment to another person can be enhanced by time.

> Love surfeits not, Lust like a glutton dies.[d]

It is a constant rebirth of surprise that the world can hold something so beyond imagination that is at the same time a familiar homecoming. It is a fullness of joy that entirely outruns any explanation in terms of the pleasure principle, or of the threat of time. Past and future unite in making the immediacy of the present moment what it is.

> . . . immediate reality is transcended in any kind of joy . . . we have to distinguish between *pleasure by release of tension,* and the *active feeling of enjoyment* and freedom so characteristic of joy. . . . Pleasure may be a necessary state of respite. But it is a phenomenon of standstill. . . . It separates us from the world and the other individuals in it; it is equilibrium, quietness. In joy there is disequilibrium . . . disequilibrium, leading toward fruitful activity and a particular kind of self-realization.[a]

Openness to relatedness with other persons and the search for self-identity are not two problems but one dialectical process; as one finds more relatedness to other persons one discovers more of oneself; as the sense of one's own identity becomes clearer and more firmly rooted one can more completely go out to others. It is not a loss of oneself, an "impoverishment," but a way of finding more of oneself when one means most to others whom one has chosen. Nor must complete finding of oneself, as Fromm and others sometimes seem to imply, precede finding oneself in and through other persons. Identity is never wholly realized. Love is never perfect. Strength to apprehend love that is beyond anxiety, beyond the need to use other persons for one's own security, beyond desire for power over others is never complete, but may grow throughout life. Like identity and mutuality with others it is a lifetime process of discovery.

> . . . in the struggle for existence in a world ruled by anxiety . . . the surrender to the . . . experience of Love appears softening and therefore weakening. . . . Love is deeply taboo. . . . Sex without love belongs in the sphere of power operations. . . . In the transcendence of Love there is no . . . struggle for self-assertion, for in the we-ness the Self is received as a gift of grace. . . . The fight for right, entitlement . . . becomes superfluous, for . . . Love experiences space as bountiful, infinite. . . .[b]

Love increasingly transcends power, anxiety, and shame. A person who cannot love cannot reveal himself. Exposure in love is beneficent.

USES OF LANGUAGE

The importance for developing a sense of one's own identity of language and of communication has appeared throughout these pages. It is hard to know whether to discuss language as a subdivision of communication or communication as a subdivision of language. Each way of statement expresses a truth: communication has many other forms than language, particularly if the term language is confined to verbal expression; language has many uses beyond, not only the conveying of information, but even beyond communication.* I use language here as the more inclusive term to stress the varieties of discovery it makes possible beyond communication with other persons; but this is not intended to minimize the importance of the varieties of nonverbal communication.

Each of the manifold uses of language has its special importance for the discovery of identity: the very acquisition of speech is a major factor in helping a child to know who he is and in opening to him a new field of exploration and enjoyment—language itself.†

Language also helps to organize for the individual his perceptions of the world. Without going as far as the statement of the Sapir-Whorf hypothesis that what we call the real world is to a large extent the creation of the language habits of the social

* Contrast Whatmough's italicized statement that "*Language is first and foremost a means of transmitting information*" (*Language*, p. 12) and his statement that "communication is identical in purpose and subject matter whether it is face to face, or over the telephone or radio, or by telegraph." (*Ibid.*, p. 209.)

† Cf. pp. 171-81 and Erikson's statement that ". . . a child who is learning to speak . . . is acquiring one of the prime functions supporting a sense of individual autonomy. . . . The mere indication of an ability to give intentional sound-signs immediately obligates the child to "*say* what he wants". . . . Speech not only commits him to the kind of voice he has and to the mode of speech he develops; it also *defines him* as one responded to by those around him. . . . Furthermore, a spoken word is a pact. . . . This intrinsic relationship of speech . . . to the social value of verbal commitment and uttered truth is strategic among the experiences which support (or fail to support) a sound ego development." ("The Problem of Ego Identity," *Journal of the American Psychoanalytic Association*, Vol. IV, No. 1, Jan. 1956, p. 70.)

group,* we must, nevertheless, recognize that language is, at the very least, a selective factor in helping to determine what we perceive and what we emphasize in that perception—what we experience. Not only is what we can express and communicate inevitably determined by what we experience, but what we perceive and experience is in part determined by the modes of expression available to us. Around what aspects of experience shall we draw a circle, separating them out by the ascription of a word? And shall that word be a noun, a verb, or an adjective? How shall we organize and classify the flood of our perceptions? How was Darwin to go about classifying the unfamiliar phenomena that he saw to his amazement on the voyage of the *Beagle*? Why does Aaron Copland in trying to explain to the layman *What to Listen for in Music*[a] list the four separate "elements" in music as Rhythm, Melody, Harmony, and Tone Color and then add Musical Texture and Musical Structure? There might be other ways of naming and classifying what enters into music. Such questions as these our experience and the impulse to communicate it sets for us. The language patterns available to us help to determine the ways we answer them.

Because of the manifold possible ways of describing the world about us and because of the kinds of misunderstandings that can come about from confusions in the use of words, it is natural that there have been recurrent organized efforts to have more fixity in language. The development of languages of signs that reduce differences of interpretation to a minimum has been a major factor in the growth of Western science and mathematics, and will continue to be indispensable for scientific discoveries and for exchange of scientific information among peoples.

But the question that has been raised repeatedly in this discussion is whether, with all the gains, there may also be a loss in concentration on a language of signs of unequivocal meaning. The detachment of science may, if emphasized at the expense of

* See pp. 171-81 for discussion of the Sapir-Whorf hypothesis and for Whatmough's and Feuer's criticism of it.

other relations to the world, bring an impoverishment of experience, and in so far as it is an inadequate account of the world, a distortion of science as well. For the sake of what we can perceive and experience as well as of what we can communicate it is important to search the possibilities of language beyond the language of unequivocal signs.

From a number of widely different fields, including that of language in the limited sense of verbal communication, there comes evidence of willingness to take the risks involved in going beyond fixed signs in order to reach kinds of experiences, kinds of discoveries, and kinds of communication otherwise impossible. Words are sometimes sensitive instruments of precision with which delicate operations may be performed and swift, elusive truths may be touched; often they are clumsy tools with which we grope in the dark toward truths more inaccessible but no less significant.

The special contributions of Gestalt psychology to the expanded possibilities of language have been mentioned earlier. Arnheim's insistence that expression (that is, total emotional content) is more primary in perceptual experience than data of color, shape, sound, opens the way to recognition of the significance of finding means of communicating such experience.[b]

In therapy, Frieda Fromm-Reichmann, Marguerite Sechehaye, and others have patiently and imaginatively let go of the more familiar sign languages and codifications of psychoanalysis in order to discover through what symbols they might establish communication with schizophrenics.* Their work opens up extraordinary possibilities of entering with new perceptions into the lives of other persons whose illness cuts them off from social relations, and of finding ways of re-establishing communication with them.[c] If discovery of symbols of communication is possible in extreme mental illness, it suggests that greater search for such symbols might be valuable in psychoanalytic therapy with persons less seriously ill, in teaching, and between persons who are trying to understand each other.

In art, there is an ever-renewed attempt to create the emblems that will represent reality in terms that most truly

* See p. 157.

express the perception of a particular time. "Cezanne," says Joseph Kahnweiler, "wanted to express the whole of his sensation [and] his spontaneous emotion . . . which took in the objects illuminated . . . with their volume and their position in space. In addition he wished to preserve in his pictures all those accidental modifications of the appearance of objects which are caused by light." [a] Kahnweiler describes the development since 1910 of what he calls a new factor in painting: the introduction of several views of the same object juxtaposed in one picture intended to be seen simultaneously and to compose together a single object in the eyes of the spectator.[b]

Writers of the last half-century have engaged—as writers always have in one form or another—in the hazards involved in the development of symbols, abundant with meaning, which inform the subject with a wealth of treasured experience. They employ, not signals that serve as a shorthand for a specific, limited phenomenon, but symbols that carry in themselves the antithetical sense of primal words, the multifariousness, the richness, and versatility that enlarge the possibilities of language and of experience itself. D. H. Lawrence never hesitated to make a fool of himself in experimenting with the verbal symbols that would most fully convey his meaning. Joyce and Virginia Woolf broke through all established canons in the same endeavor. Leo Spitzer says of Cervantes—one of the greatest artists and prophets in extending the range of language—"What, ultimately, is offered here [in *Don Quijote*] is a criticism of the arbitrariness of any fixed expression in human language." Spitzer believes that later artists influenced by Cervantes, among whom he includes Gide, Proust, Joyce, and Woolf, have failed to appreciate the full richness and unity of his "perspectivism" in use of language and its relation to culture.[c]

Among contemporary critics William Empson has given most specific attention to ambiguity and manifold meaning in words, as well as to the part that rhythm and sound play in determining structure of language. Using the materials of English poetry and prose he has elaborately demonstrated that words and syntactical structures that include both or all parts of a relationship, that give expression to surplus meaning, are actually more precise and more objective than those that designate only one part. Tracing, for example, the multifarious histories and meanings that enter into the use of "honest" in *Othello,* of "fool" in Erasmus' *Praise of Folly* and in *King Lear,* of "sense" in *Measure for Measure,* he makes it clear that we are not being exact, accurate, or precise, or in any sense getting at the truth of what we are dealing with if we do not take into full account the ambiguity, the complexity, and the surplus meaning that are the essence of these words.[a]

T. S. Eliot says of his composition: "I know that a poem or a section of a poem tends to appear first in the shape of a rhythm before developing into words,* and that this rhythm is capable of giving birth to the idea and the image." [b]

Even in mathematics, often used as the model for a language of signs, Jacques Hadamard describes the necessity of going beyond a sign language for creative discovery. He says that for himself a mathematical concept must first be grasped as "one global idea," a mental image or picture, before it can be expressed in words or in mathematical signs.[c] He describes his use of "a strange and cloudy imagery" in arriving at a new mathematical proof, and says:

> I need a mechanism in order to have a simultaneous view of all elements of the argument . . . to . . . give the problem its physiognomy.
>
> For B. O. Koopman, 'images have a symbolic rather than a diagrammatic relation to the mathematical ideas.'
>
> . . . I think . . . and so will a majority of scientific men, that the more complicated and difficult a question is, the more we distrust words, the more we feel we must control that dangerous ally and *its sometimes treacherous precision.*[d] (Italics mine.)

Norbert Wiener has testified to similar experience.

> [The rewards of mathematics] are of exactly the same character as those of the artist. To see a difficult, uncompromising material take

* Cf. C. P. Snow, "Dickens at Work" on Dickens' "mastery over a first design" of a novel before he could begin work. ". . . this grasp of complex material, a grasp both passionate and articulated, was, perhaps his most unusual gift." (*New Statesman and Nation,* July 27, 1957.)

living shape and meaning is to be a Pygmalion, whether the material is stone or hard, stone-like logic. . . . The great strain on memory in mathematical work is for me not so much the retention of a vast mass of fact . . . as of *the simultaneous aspects of the particular problem on which I have been working* and of *the conversion of my fleeting impressions into something permanent* enough to have a place in memory. For I have found that if I have been able to cram all my past ideas of what the problem really involves into *a single comprehensive impression,* the problem is more than half solved.[a] (Italics mine.)

In his study of "Memory and Childhood Amnesia" [b] Schachtel gives a particularly illuminating account of the way in which language inevitably reflects the dominant preoccupations and the limitations of a society. By such reflection it restricts perception and experience unless refreshed by innovation. Certain kinds of experience may be buried or lost because the culture provides no language through which they can be expressed. He dissents from Freud's view that early childhood experiences are forgotten because they are so largely concerned with sexual desires later repressed or censored. He advances the hypothesis that these experiences are forgotten because they are of an immediate and diffused nature for which the categories and verbal signs of the conventional adult world, notably in contemporary Western society, provide no means of expression.* As the child becomes more socialized he becomes less capable of entering fully and vividly into the kinds of experiences that were open to him earlier, and, since customary verbal categories are unsuitable, less able to lay hold of any media of recall.

. . . the . . . categories of memory . . . are not suitable vehicles to receive and reproduce experiences of the quality and intensity typical of early childhood. The world of modern Western civilization has no use for this type of experience . . . it cannot permit the memory of it, because *such memory . . . would explode the restrictive social order of this civilization.*[c] (Italics mine.)

* Korzybski notes that magicians find children more difficult to deceive than others because they are not habituated to conventional seeing. ("Language in the Perceptual Process," in Blake and Ramsey, *Perception: An Approach to Personality*, p. 200.)

Adult memory reflects life as a road with occasional sign-posts and milestones rather than as the landscape through which this road has led. . . . The capacity to see and feel what is there gives way to the tendency to see and feel what one expects to see and feel, which, in turn, is what one is expected to see and feel because everybody else does. Experience increasingly assumes the form of the cliche under which it will be recalled because this cliché is what conventionally is remembered by others.[a]

That part of the experience which transcends the memory schema as performed by the culture is in danger of being lost because there exists as yet no vessel . . . in which to preserve it.[b]

The innovator, poet, artist, scientist, or political revolutionary attempts to recreate the capacity to perceive and to communicate diffused, whole experiences, to give form to experiences that have the intensity and immediacy of the child's perception of the world.

The artist, the writer, the poet, if they have any real claim to their vocation, must be capable of non-schematic experience. They must be perceptive; that is, they must experience, see, hear, feel things in a way which somewhere transcends the cultural, conventional experience schemata. The relative freedom from these experience schemata is also freedom, to whatever extent, from the conventional memory schemata. . . . One might say that the normal amnesia, that which people usually are unable to recall, is an illuminating index to the quality of any given culture and society.[c]

The profound difficulties Schachtel describes in finding a medium for recalling and expressing deep autobiographical experiences are sometimes more easily surmounted by the use of the third person in an art form. This provides at once a sense of newness, as if a diffused sensory experience were being felt for the first time in an uncodified form in describing the experience of a person other than oneself, and protection against painful exposure in the attempt to recall a particularly wounding experience in one's own past. There is a question whether such revelations as those to be found in *Of Human Bondage, The Way of All Flesh, The Mill on the Floss, Strait Is the Gate,* may not at times succeed in giving more detail of the nuance of tone, gesture, and feeling than more openly autobiographical confessions.* Joyce in *Stephen Hero* recognizes that such use of dramatic roles sometimes allows more recall and revelation than would be possible in a first-person autobiographical statement.[a]

In all of these fields innovators are trying out new ways of perceiving, reshaping, and expressing reality. They stress, not a lineal approach, but proportion, relations, variability, the perception of phenomena both from within and from without. All these attempts to take the risks involved in discovering or creating new ways of experience and of communication have direct bearing on shame and the sense of identity.

It is not only that there is no adequate language of shame, of identity, of the deepest experiences of mutual joy and grief. The present theoretical and pragmatic acceptance of aggression, prestige, and power as central springs of action put still other barriers in the way of experiencing and communicating shame, joy, love, wonder, curiosity, sense of honor, and desire for significance beyond recognized achievement. Lack of a language contributes to the sense of estrangement. If, however, one can sufficiently risk uncovering oneself and sufficiently trust another person, to seek means of communicating shame, the risking of exposure can be in itself an experience of release, expansion, self-revelation, a coming forward of belief in oneself, and entering into the mind and feeling of another person.

It may be asked why, since the language of intimacy will always be to a large extent a language of gesture, facial expression, and touch, it should be important to enlarge the possibilities of verbal language for such communication. For at least three reasons: 1. Lack of a verbal means of communication of certain experiences may sometimes lead to atrophy or lack of awareness of the experiences themselves. 2. Ranges of mutual exploration may be cut off and unnecessary misunderstandings may arise if there is a feeling that words should not be used or an unwillingness to search for words to use as one medium of communication. 3. The creation of symbols in language is a

* Within a family or other close relation of intimacy, the use of banter or joking nicknames may serve a somewhat similar function of recall, or of expressing and at the same time veiling tenderness, which might for some persons involve a kind of shame if expressed more directly.

characteristically human ability that can bring unconscious creative forces into relation with conscious effort, subject into relation with object, can give form to hitherto unknown things and hence make possible the apprehension of new truth.

A kind of moral obligation is involved in extending the depth of experience and in communicating experience as fully (which is another way of saying as accurately) as possible. Such communication necessitates the discovery and the creation of symbols that can express deep insight. This obligation is particularly that of the artist. But every individual engages in the process of gradually making the distinction between the self that is in here and the world that is out there. This separation is never complete. One can become, and continue to be, oneself only through discovering and rediscovering ways of distinction from and communication with other persons as well as the nonpersonal world. The distinction and the communication are parts of one process, each essential to the other. Only a language of symbol, of paradox, of abundant meaning can communicate the deeper and more elusive ranges of human experience.

SHAME AND PRIDE

To suggest that in order to approach the questions Who am I? Where do I belong? men should live beyond prescribed codes, in terms of the multiple possibilities of their period of history, and that they should create symbols to enlarge the meaning of life is to say that they should commit the sin of pride. They should seek to become like gods, themselves knowing good and evil. They should "stretch a crumme of dust from heav'n to hell." Nothing is so ridiculous or involves such risk as this.

What may one venture to say of man's humility and man's pride—the theme of Aeschylus, of the authors of Job, of Blake, of Goethe? Nothing, perhaps, except that many contemporary psychological concepts tend to deny or to dwarf the problem, and that it is an enduring human problem that cannot be diminished. The emerging ways of studying personality described do not answer or offer any promise of answers to such major problems. Rather, they clarify errors of reductionism and omission, point out inadequacies in our thinking, and permit us to approach nearer only to realize more fully the immensities we confront.* When we ask the ultimate questions, whether about the direction of our own lives or about the meaning of existence, the outcome of thinking is not an answer but a transformed way of thinking, not propositions to assent to but heightened power of apprehension.

Whatever changes may take place in the social order so that it becomes more favorable to expression of diverse human possibilities, the tragic limitations of man's fate remain. Any search for identity that ignores them is taking place in a meager or in an unreal world. It is only with full awareness of these necessities that men can transform shame, affirm their pride, and continue their search for significance. "The greatest mystery," says Malraux, "is not that we should have been thrown up by chance between the profusion of matter and the profusion of the stars, but that, in that prison, we should be able to get out of ourselves images sufficiently powerful to deny our insignificance."

But the tragic inevitabilities that surround men's lives are not their only tragedies. What part of the scriptural account does Blake select as a basis for depicting the tragedy of the Crucifixion? The drawing shows the backs of the three crosses. Behind them—untouched by the light from the Cross—greedy, rapacious men cast dice for the garments of Christ.[a]

The existentialist stress on the inevitable isolation and homelessness of man, and on death as the most important fact in life, tends to minimize, not only positive affirmations of joy and courage,† but the processes of history and the varying possibilities in different concrete historical situations. "Our natural and *social* environment oppresses us with its foreignness, its unsuit-

* Morris Cohen, commenting on the philosophy of Hoernlé and Bosanquet in a letter to Justice Holmes, August 7, 1920, said, "Starting with the assumption that everything is ultimately known or knowable, they cannot possibly do much for the genuine extension of the realm of human knowledge." (Felix Cohen, ed., "The Holmes-Cohen Correspondence," *Journal of the History of Ideas,* Vol. IX, No. 1, Jan. 1948, p. 20.) Cohen is by no means preaching subjectivism. It does not mean that man can know nothing because he cannot know everything.

† This is not true of Paul Tillich and of some phases of existentialism.

ability as a home for all that is specifically human about us as individuals. If we are genuine persons, sensitive to the human situation, we can gain no hold or support in nature or *society*." [a] (Italics mine.) It is not necessary to be blind to the limits that surround life to believe that changes in the social situation can bring about some changes in the realization of human possibilities, and that within the necessities significance may be found. History continues to be an attempt by man to make a home for himself in the world, and philosophy a heightened interest in life, not a trained indifference to life.

How is the search for significance to be carried on? And what is the relation between the kind of pride it involves and shame and the sense of identity?

Pride is often contrasted with shame. Shame and pride, in this view, are regarded as opposites; shame is the response to scorn or ridicule from an audience; pride is self-aggrandizement in response to acclaim or approval by an audience. It is clear from all that has been said that I share Schilder's belief that such use of Platonic opposites in regard to shame and pride (or any other concepts) is fruitless and misleading. This use of shame and pride, furthermore, conceives both too narrowly, and fails to recognize the range of experiences of shame that has been suggested in these pages and to distinguish among different kinds of pride.

Pride that is arrogance and satisfaction in power and superiority over others often arises from a sense of oneself as contemptible, ridiculous, or dishonorable.[b] It depends on external approval and has constantly to be reinforced. It does not have sustaining quality.

Pride as arrogance the Greeks called *hubris*. It was overweening, a contempt for men and a defiance of the gods, which brought an inevitable tragic outcome. Very different is the Greek *philotimo*, which is honor, inviolability, freedom in oneself through selective identifications with aspects of one's own or a wider culture. If one has *philotimo*, self-respect, then *hubris*, arrogance in relation to others, becomes unnecessary.[c]

Tragedy may be the outcome of pride based on insecurity and desire for self-aggrandizement and of pride based on confidence in human possibilities, but these are very different tragic outcomes. The tragedy of Macbeth has elements of meanness and need of constant external reinforcement, that of Prometheus or of Oedipus partakes of grandeur since man overreaches himself.*

In the medieval world pride of any sort was one of the seven deadly sins, an impiety toward God, whose punishment was sure. The Reformation restated the paradox of pride. No one has been more eloquent on the sin of pride and the nothingness and worthlessness of man before God than Calvin; yet emphasis on the trust of man in his individual conscience can lead to the pride of questioning the authority of any religious or secular institution.

For some persons pride that has its roots in self-respect is an impossibility, and even the idea of such self-regard is incredible. Iago did not believe that anyone could have such a feeling toward himself.

> . . . since I could distinguish betwixt a benefit and an injury, I never found man that knew how to love himself.[a]

Mr. Casaubon knew only the more limiting sort of pride based on the feeling of insecurity.

> . . . the idea of calling forth a show of compassion by frankly admitting an alarm or a sorrow was necessarily intolerable to him. Every proud mind knows something of this experience, and perhaps it is only to be overcome by a sense of fellowship deep enough to make all efforts at isolation seem mean and petty instead of exalting.
>
> . . . [The] most characteristic result [of Mr. Casaubon's hard intellectual labors] was . . . a morbid consciousness that others did not give him the place which he had not demonstrably merited . . . and a passionate resistance to the confession that he had achieved nothing.

* Cf. Joseph Campbell's account of pride in his description of the mythological hero: "The tyrant is proud, and therein resides his doom. He is proud because he thinks of his strength as his own; thus he is in the clown role, as a mistaker of shadow for substance; it is his destiny to be tricked. The mythological hero . . . brings a knowledge of the secret of the tyrant's doom. . . . The hero-deed is a continuous shattering of the crystalizations of the moment. (*The Hero with a Thousand Faces,* Pantheon Books, 1949, p. 337.)

Thus his intellectual ambition which seemed to others to have absorbed and dried him, was really no security against wounds, least of all against those which came from Dorothea.[a]

There can be a pride rooted in oneself in relation to the world that does not stand in constant need of reassurance from others or of demonstrating itself. Emily Dickinson writes:

> Unmoved—she notes the Chariots—pausing—
> At her low Gate—
> Unmoved—an Emperor be Kneeling
> Upon her Mat—

If we conceive that pride can be, not arrogance as compensation for uncertainty, but a quality of honor and self-respect, we come closer to a central, inescapable question: How can an individual reach his full stature without committing the sin of pride, attempting to reach beyond man's limitations? Or, conversely, how is it possible for an individual to acknowledge the universe as greater than himself and to humble himself before it without denying his self-respect and abasing himself as mean and insignificant? Nietzsche in the assertion of individual strength felt man allied to the universe, but for him this meant contempt for most men and for any kind of society. Fromm attacks the Calvinist conception of the worthlessness of man and regards self-respect and self-love as the basis of morality, but he does not dwell on the ways in which this is congruent with humility before the world or is related to harmony with the traditions of one's own or a wider culture.

Contemporary thought sometimes escapes the question of the relation between pride and humility by resting in irony as a substitute for confronting paradox. Irony can wear the appearance of paradox. It is a contradiction, but a logical contradiction that can be resolved, and that depends for its effect on awareness of the inseparability of the overt and the implicit parts of the ironical statement and of the possibility of their resolution. Paradox is contradiction that inheres in the nature of things. It cannot be resolved. It can only be transcended, in Hegel's terms, *aufgehoben*.

Trying to understand the relation between pride and humility brings us back to a paradox—the paradox that the more fully one is aware of his own individual identity, the more fully he is also aware of the immensity of the universe and of his place in it.* For some individuals it is deeply true that without a sense of potential significance in the world, a sense of oneself is impossible. The recurrent attempt to affirm a principle that has no immediate result, no measurable pragmatic outcome, is an affirmation of possible meaning in life, a reaffirmation of significance.

Such search for significance includes identifications, but identifications beyond those of one's immediate situation in space and time. It involves, also, efforts to expose the repressions and contradictions of present society, to find seeds of wider values in them and to engage in active efforts to change society in the direction of fuller realization. One of the sources of pride in being a human being is the ability to bear present frustrations in the interests of longer purposes.†

Search for significance takes on more hope the greater the aspects of the world with which we can identify. People differ markedly according to whether they regard the possibility of wider identifications as a threat to or an enlargement of themselves.

Some persons when they encounter a new or strange situation, idea, or person have an immediate impulse to see where it fits into their scheme of things; others invite a pause, an abeyance, to allow their view of the world to be modified or

* Cf. F. M. Cornford's contrast between Olympian morality with its emphasis on not overstepping the limits of one's allotted province and with *hybris* as the cardinal sin and Pythagorean morality with its emphasis on continuities and a way of life. (*From Religion to Philosophy*. Harper, Torchbooks, 1957, p. 181.)

† This has been implied through much of this discussion. Cf. Erikson's statement: "Man in the service of a faith can stand meaningful frustration . . . in the use of reason there lies the eternal temptation to do with human data in experiment and argument what the child does with them in play . . . to reduce them to a size and an order in which they seem manageable. Thus human data are treated as if the human being were an animal, or a machine, or a statistical item. . . . The human being up to a point is all of these things, and under certain conditions can be reduced to being nothing but their facsimiles. But the attempt to make man more exploitable by reducing him to a simpler model of himself cannot lead to an essentially human psychology." (*Childhood and Society*, Norton, 1950, pp. 373-5.)

enlarged by this new encounter. These differences are reflected in habits of speech. For an academic person who makes use of such expressions as: "Does he know *his* Ben Jonson?" "*His* medieval history?" "*His* Darwin?" "*His* Goethe?"—any event, person, or development seems to be regarded as a part of his mental world. He may be less likely to raise the question as to how he fits into a world that has been made more spacious and complex by Ben Jonson, by the Middle Ages, by Darwin, by Goethe.

Ibsen, in *The Master Builder,* depicts the different ways in which different persons relate themselves to the phenomenon of size. Schachtel says of such differences, "Standing on the top of a high mountain . . . one person feels primarily the elevation of his position . . . his self participates in the grandeur of the mountain on which he stands. Another person feels dwarfed by the grandeur of the same view, he feels lost in the vast expanse, he does not experience identification, but opposition or comparison of his small self and the gigantic world around him." [a]

The transformation of the paradox of pride in one's own identity and humility in relation to the universe would seem to consist in taking each in the large, in its full dimensions. Experiences of inappropriateness in shame may be belittling if they are simply covered with the most readily available roles or forms. They may be enlarging if placed against a more ample perspective. Such larger identifications with a group of other persons, a scientific investigation or an art form, a purpose or a belief, may become not a losing but a finding of oneself. The transcending of shame, in Hegel's sense of opposites, is not pride in response to acclaim but recognition and realization of larger identifications and of one's own identity.

This enlarged perspective is sometimes referred to as a comic frame of reference.[b] The comic in this meaning is the sense of proportion that is the outcome of taking the individual self and the world in their widest reach of all that they can be. It is the condemnation of the partial masquerading as the complete. This dialectical logic includes the romanticism of self-enlargement or self-expansion by means of successive experiments with all phases of life, and also the exposure of the limits of the efforts of man to assimilate all reality to his particular needs and purposes.[a] It shows

> . . . the perpetual error of the human mind to magnify out of proportion in the name of *all* truth or *all* civilization a *particular* set of interests or values. . . . The inexhaustible source of comedy lies in the perception and exhibition of human extravagance. All comedy achieves its effect by rendering ridiculous those ailing from the illusion of perspective. . . . The folly of drawing the whole to the scale of the part is just what the dialectical method singles out as proper food for the Comic Spirit.[b]

The relation between pride and humility cannot be resolved on the guilt axis. Job's three friends exhorted him to feel guilt before God. This, Job felt, would be belittling to God and to himself. What he felt was shame for himself and for God and the world He had created. He attempted no moral justification in terms of atonement for transgression.

> If it is a test of strength, He is surely superior!
> But if it is a [question] of justice, who can arraign Him? . . .
> I am guiltless—[c]
>
> Aye, though He slay me, I tremble not;
> For all that, I will maintain His course to His face.[d]

He could not confess guilt without diminishing himself and God. He magnified his own soul and he sought to magnify God.

This magnificat took him beyond the social codes of his three friends. Living in terms of guilt and righteousness is living in terms of the sanctions and taboos of one's immediate culture. To some extent such living is necessary for everyone. Living in terms of the confronting of shame—and allowing shame to become a revelation of oneself and of one's society—makes way for living beyond the conventions of a particular culture. It makes possible the discovery of an integrity that is peculiarly one's own and of those characteristically human qualities that are at the same time most individualizing and most universal.

Pride in the sense of self-respect transcends shame, but is fully consonant with humility. Only the man with true pride in his capacities as a human being can have a significant humility; only the truly humble in apprehending the immensity of the universe and the world beyond himself can have a significant pride—a sense of his own identity.

Notes, Acknowledgments, and Index

Notes

The number preceding each note indicates the page on which the reference appears.

13[a] See Georg Misch, *A History of Autobiography in Antiquity,* Harvard University Press, 1951, Vol. I, p. 67. Misch uses the phrase "discovery of individuality."

14[a] Erik H. Erikson, *Childhood and Society,* Norton, 1950, pp. 242, 239.

15[a] Gardner Murphy, *An Introduction to Psychology,* Harper, 1951, p. 405.

16[a] Virginia Woolf, *A Writer's Diary,* Harcourt, Brace, 1954, p. 100.

16[b] See Ernest Schachtel, "Memory and Childhood Amnesia," in Patrick Mullahy, ed., *A Study of Interpersonal Relations,* Hermitage Press, 1950, for discussion of such experiences.

18[a] "Achievement expectation" is Talcott Parsons' term (*The Social System,* Free Press, 1951); the "performance principle" is used by Herbert Marcuse (*Eros and Civilization: A Philosophical Inquiry into Freud,* Beacon Press, 1955); the "success norm" is used by C. Wright Mills (*White Collar,* Oxford University Press, 1951) and by many other writers; the term "market-place psychology" is used particularly by Erich Fromm (*Escape from Freedom,* Farrar and Rinehart, 1941; *Man for Himself,* Rinehart, 1947).

21[a] Sigmund Freud, "Further Remarks on the Defence Neuro-psychoses" (1896), *Collected Papers,* Hogarth Press and The Institute of Psychoanalysis, 1950, Vol. I, p. 165.

21[b] Ruth Benedict, *The Chrysanthemum and the Sword: Patterns of Japanese Culture,* Houghton Mifflin, 1946, pp. 222 ff. and throughout. See also her *Patterns of Culture,* Houghton Mifflin, 1934.

21[c] See, for example, Francis L. Hsu, "Suppression Versus Repression," *Psychiatry,* Vol. 12, No. 3, Aug. 1949; E. R. Dodds, *The Greeks and the Irrational,* University of California Press, 1951; Talcott Parsons and Edward A. Shils, eds., *Toward a General Theory of Action,* Harvard University Press, 1951, p. 142; Margaret Mead, "Social Change and Cultural Surrogates," in Clyde Kluckhohn and Henry A. Murray, eds., *Personality in Nature, Society, and Culture,* 2d ed., Knopf, 1953, p. 658, and "Anthropological Considerations Concerning Guilt," in Martin L. Reymert, ed., *Feelings and Emotions,* McGraw-Hill, 1950, pp. 367-8.

Herman Numberg believes that guilt is directly associated with the Oedipus situation and that the feeling of guilt and the need for punishment have common roots, but that shame and feelings of inferiority are often associated with guilt. ("The Feeling of Guilt," *Psychoanalytic Quarterly,* Vol. III, No. 4, Oct. 1934, pp. 589-604.) Theodor Reik emphasizes the relation of guilt to the Oedipus myth and the myth of the fall and redemption of man and to the need for punishment. (*Dogma and Compulsion,* International Universities Press, 1951 and *Myth and Guilt,* George Braziller, 1957.)

David P. Ausubel questions the interpretations Benedict and other anthropologists make of particular behavior and particular cultures as being primarily oriented in terms of shame or guilt, but he maintains the basic distinction that shame relies on external sanctions alone, in contrast to guilt which relies also on internal sanctions. ("Relationships between Shame and Guilt in the Socializing Process," *Psychological Review,* Vol. 62, No. 5, Sept. 1955, pp. 378-90.)

22[a] I am indebted to a comment by Herbert C. Kelman for this distinction. It appears in a somewhat different form in Kurt Riezler, "Comment on the Social Psychology of Shame," *The American Journal of Sociology,* Vol. XLVIII, No. 4, Jan. 1943.

22[b] Erikson notes that Freud made little use of the concept of a self-ideal and that Freudians have tended too easily to subsume "self-ideal" under "superego." ("Ego Development and Historical Change," in *The Psychoanalytic Study of the Child,* International Universities Press, Vol. II, 1946, p. 363.) In "On Narcissism" (1914) however, Freud referred to the "ideal ego" which replaces as an object of self-love the real ego of childhood. (*Collected Papers,* Vol. IV, p. 51.)

22[c] See Franz Alexander, *Fundamentals of Psychoanalysis: A Psychoanalytic and a Cultural Study,* Norton, 1948, and "Remarks about the Relation of Inferiority Feelings to Guilt Feelings," *International Journal of Psychoanalysis,* Vol. XIX, Part I, Jan. 1938.

22[d] Max Scheler, for example, finds the essential characteristic of shame to be conflict between man's spiritual powers and his servitude to his body. He speaks of a bridge or passage between these two orders of being that is essential for man in order for him to be human. This is shame rooted in the nature of man, not in a particular culture. (*La Pudeur,* trans. from the German by M. Dupuy, Paris, Editions Montaigne, 1952.) See also Eckhard J. Koehle, "Personality: A Study According to the Philosophies of Value and Spirit of Max Scheler and Nicolai Hartman," unpublished Ph.D. dissertation, Columbia University, 1941.

Arnold Isenberg believes that shame is best understood in its relation to pride, that shame is related to feelings of weakness or inferiority and that, although the disfavor of others usually enters into feelings of shame, there is some evidence for the existence of sources of shame independent of society. ("Natural Pride and Natural Shame," *Philosophy and Phenomenological Research,* Vol. X, No. 1, Sept. 1949, pp. 8, 12.)

22[e] Gerhart Piers and Milton B. Singer, *Shame and Guilt,* Charles C. Thomas, 1953, p. 11.

22[f] Franz Alexander, *Fundamentals of Psychoanalysis,* pp. 123, 127. Cf. Irwin Katz, "Emotional Expression in Failure," *Journal of Abnormal and Social Psychology,* Vol. 45, No. 2, Apr. 1950, pp. 329-49. Dorothy Lee takes a position somewhat similar to Alexander's. Shame, in her view, goes deeper than guilt, and this contrast is recognized by Greeks, Syrians, and other peoples for whom "They" or "The Others" are not as separate as in our society. (Personal communication, 1951.)

22[g] See, especially, Alexander, "Remarks about the Relation of Inferiority Feelings to Guilt Feelings."

24[a] Riezler, "Comment on the Social Psychology of Shame." See also his *Man: Mutable and Immutable,* Henry Regnery, 1951.

24[b] Riezler, "Comment on the Social Psychology of Shame," p. 462.

24[c] *Ibid.,* p. 463. Werner Jaeger notes that Democritus added to the concept of *aidos* the idea of shame that a man feels not before the law but before himself. (*Paideia: The Ideals of Greek Culture,* Oxford University Press, 1939, Vol. I, pp. 327-8.)

24[d] Zephaniah 3:5.

25[a] *The Winter's Tale,* III, ii, 85-6.

25[b] *Henry VI,* Part III, II, ii, 145. In view of the apparently close connection between shame and self it is interesting to note that the old word self was not compounded as a prefix in English until the late sixteenth and early seventeenth centuries. (Logan Pearsall Smith, *The English Language,* Home University Library, 1912, pp. 236-7.)

25[c] Riezler, "Comment on the Social Psychology of Shame," p. 462.

25[d] Deuteronomy 19:13; 21:9. (Concordance based on the King James version.) Sin and trespass sometimes occur as possible synonyms of guilt.

25[e] Genesis 26:10; Psalms 51:14.

25[f] Psalms 4:2.

25[g] Philippians 3:19.

25[h] Psalms 40:14.
25[i] Jeremiah 51:51.
25[j] Acts 5:41.
25[k] Hebrews 12:2.
25[l] *Bartlett's Concordance.*
26[a] *Henry IV,* Part I, III, i, 62.
26[b] *King John,* I, i, 64.
26[c] *Richard II,* V, iii, 67-71.
26[d] *Henry VI,* Part III, III, iii, 184-5.
26[e] *Pericles,* IV, iii, 23.
26[f] On this point see John Dover Wilson, *The Fortunes of Falstaff,* Macmillan, 1944, pp. 70-2. Cf. also William Empson's discussion of Shakespeare's use of "honour" and "honest" in *The Structure of Complex Words,* Chatto and Windus, 1951, Chaps. 9, 10, 11.
28[a] W. Somerset Maugham, *Of Human Bondage,* Modern Library, p. 47.
28[b] Quoted in Aileen Pippett, *The Moth and the Star,* Little, Brown, 1955, pp. 108, 323-4.
28[c] Rousseau, *Confessions,* Modern Library, pp. 88-9.
29[a] Tolstoy, *Anna Karenina,* Modern Library, p. 95. (All page references to *Anna Karenina* are to the Modern Library edition, but in some cases Nathan Haskell Dole's and Louise and Aylmer Maude's translations are used when they seem more revealing than Constance Garnett's translation.)
29[b] *Ibid.,* p. 119.
29[c] Dostoyevsky, *The Brothers Karamazov,* Modern Library, p. 587.
29[d] "'A Child Is Being Beaten'" (1919), *Collected Papers,* Vol. II, p. 172.
30[a] *Of Human Bondage,* p. 47.
30[b] *Anna Karenina,* p. 119.
30[c] *Ibid.,* p. 131.
30[d] *Ibid.,* p. 176.
31[a] *Ibid.,* p. 342.
31[b] *Ibid.,* p. 179.
31[c] *Ibid.,* p. 263.
31[d] *Notes from the Underground* in *The Short Novels of Dostoevsky,* Dial Press, 1945, p. 184.
31[e] Nathaniel Hawthorne, *The Scarlet Letter,* Houghton Mifflin, Riverside Press, p. 85. See also the reference to "the child of its father's guilt and its mother's shame." (*Ibid.,* p. 141.)
32[a] W. H. Auden in the *New Yorker,* Dec. 18, 1954, pp. 142-3.
32[b] Cf. Paul Schilder on the importance of the image of one's own body, *Image and Appearance of the Human Body,* Kegan Paul, Trench, Trubner, 1935; Erikson, *Childhood and Society,* p. 224; and Kurt Goldstein's discussion of anxiety as something that "gets at us from the back . . . coming from no particular place," in "The

Effect Of Brain Damage On The Personality," *Psychiatry*, Vol. 15, No. 3, Aug. 1952, p. 256.

Cf. also James Rae, "On Shame," *Journal of Mental Science*, Vol. 62, No. 259, Oct. 1916, pp. 756-7: ". . . physical signs and accompaniments of shame . . . [show] a confusion of thought. . . . To exhibit the extreme of grief the Greek artist painted a curtain to conceal the face as if from shame at revealing emotion."

32[c] Franz Kafka, *The Trial*, Knopf, 1937, pp. 27, 84, 10, 79, 199.

33[a] See, for example, Agnes Keith, *Three Came Home*, Michael Joseph, 1948.

33[b] Joost A. M. Meerloo, *The Rape of the Mind: The Psychology of Thought Control, Menticide, and Brainwashing*, World Publishing Co., 1956, p. 75. Cf. also *ibid.*, p. 91, and William Sargant, *Battle for the Mind: A Physiology of Conversion and Brain-washing*, Heinemann, 1957.

33[c] Psalms 34:5.

33[d] Ezra 9:6.

33[e] Jeremiah 6:15.

33[f] *Henry VI*, Part I, II, iv, 64-7.

33[g] *King Lear*, IV, ii, 62-3.

34[a] *Anna Karenina*, p. 62.

34[b] *Ibid.*, p. 224.

34[c] *Ibid.*, p. 377.

34[d] See Max Scheler, *La Pudeur*, throughout.

34[e] *Childhood and Society*, p. 223, and "On the Sense of Inner Identity," in Robert P. Knight and Cyrus R. Friedman, eds., *Psychoanalytic Psychiatry and Psychology: Clinical and Theoretical Papers*, Austen Riggs Center, Vol. I, International Universities Press, 1954, p. 355.

35[a] George Bernard Shaw, *Selected Prose*, Dodd, Mead, 1952, p. 35. The finding of a place in society that is accepted by others is related to the Chinese concept of being "in face." Erving Goffman has discussed this concept in relation to feelings of inferiority and shame. "When a person senses that he is in face he typically responds with feelings of confidence and assurance. . . . [If he feels in wrong face or out of face he is] likely to feel ashamed and inferior . . . [he] had relied upon the encounter to support an image of self to which he had become emotionally attached and which he now finds threatened." ("On Face-Work," *Psychiatry*, Vol. 18, No. 3, Aug. 1955, p. 214.)

36[a] Mark Twain, *Huckleberry Finn*, Harper, 1923, pp. 126-32.

36[b] See, for example, Kurt Riezler, "Comment on the Social Psychology of Shame"; Arnold Isenberg, "Natural Pride and Natural Shame"; Max Scheler, *La Pudeur*.

37[a] Cf. Franz Alexander's statement that feelings of inferiority and inadequacy, unlike feelings of guilt, are not connected with any sense of justice. ("Remarks about the Relation of Inferiority Feelings to Guilt Feelings," p. 44.)

37[b] Cf. Anselm Strauss, *An Essay on Identity* (mimeographed), University of Chicago, 1957, p. 128.

38[a] From *Der Rosenkavalier.*

38[b] *King Lear,* I, iv, 318-21.

38[c] *Ibid.,* III, ii, 19-20.

38[d] *Ibid.,* IV, vi, 109.

39[a] *Notes from the Underground,* p. 207.

39[b] *A Writer's Diary,* p. 223.

39[c] *Anna Karenina,* p. 120.

40[a] *Ibid.,* p. 129.

40[b] *Ibid.,* p. 109.

40[c] Joseph Conrad, *Chance,* Doubleday, Doran, 1914, p. 223.

40[d] Honoré de Balzac, *Père Goriot,* Modern Library, p. 18.

40[e] Jean de la Bruyère, *Les "Caractères" de Théophraste,* Librairie Larousse, 1949, Vol. II.

40[f] V. S. Pritchett, review of Virginia Woolf, *The Captain's Death Bed and Other Essays, New Statesman and Nation,* May 13, 1950.

41[a] *Anna Karenina,* pp. 178-9.

41[b] *The Eternal Husband* in *The Short Novels of Dostoevsky,* p. 354.

41[c] Dostoyevsky, *The Devils (The Possessed),* Penguin, 1953, pp. 66, 191-2, 305.

41[d] Dostoyevsky, *The Idiot,* Penguin, 1955.

42[a] William Faulkner, *Light in August,* Modern Library, 1933, pp. 168-87.

42[b] *Père Goriot,* p. 80. Cf. T. S. Eliot's discussion of Hamlet's emotion as "exceeding its object." ("Hamlet" in *Selected Essays,* Faber and Faber, 1932, pp. 145-6.) One may disagree with Eliot's interpretation of Hamlet and still recognize the importance of the kind of emotional discrepancy he describes.

42[c] Robert K. Merton has suggested this view as a possibility.

42[d] This classification has been suggested by Herbert C. Kelman.

43[a] Freud, *The Psychopathology of Everyday Life,* in A. A. Brill, *The Basic Writings of Sigmund Freud,* Modern Library, 1938.

43[b] Job 6:20. (Jastrow translation.)

45[a] Aldous Huxley, *Point Counter Point,* Doubleday, Doran, 1928, p. 72.

45[b] Turgenev, *A House of Gentlefolk,* Macmillan, 1906, pp. 154-5.

45[c] Cf. Erikson, *Childhood and Society,* p. 219 and throughout.

45[d] Ernest Schachtel, "The Development of Focal Attention and the Emergence of Reality," *Psychiatry,* Vol. 17, No. 4, Nov. 1954, pp. 313-6.

46[a] George Eliot, *The Mill on the Floss,* Harper Library Edition, p. 136.

47[a] *Othello,* III, iii, 19.

47[b] George Madden Martin, *Emmy Lou, Her Book and Her Heart.* Copyright 1902 by McClure, Phillip and Company, reprinted by permission of Doubleday & Company, Inc., pp. 6-8.

48[a] *Ibid.,* pp. 56-60.

48[b] Norbert Wiener, *Ex-Prodigy: My Childhood and Youth,* Simon and Schuster, 1953, pp. 81-2.

49[a] Rainer Maria Rilke, *The Journal of My Other Self,* trans. by M. O. Herter Norton and John Linton, Norton, 1930, pp. 138-9.

49[b] This collapse of trust in other people and in their interpretations of the world is, Hilde Lewinsky believes, an essential element in shyness. It results in inhibition that is not volitional, but compulsory, a feeling of not being wanted, a fear of being misunderstood, of being an outsider, mistrusting one's power to understand what is told him. ("The Nature of Shyness," *British Journal of Psychology,* Vol. 32, Part 2, Oct. 1941, pp. 105-06.)

50[a] Jean-Paul Sartre, *Being and Nothingness: An Essay on Phenomenological Ontology,* trans. by Hazel E. Barnes, Philosophical Library, 1956, p. 221. See also pp. 235, 237, 249, 364, 368, 377. Sartre says, "the Other is the indispensable mediator between myself and me. I am ashamed of myself *as I appear* to the Other." (*Ibid.,* p. 222.) See also Erikson, "The Problem of Ego Identity," *Journal of the American Psychoanalytic Association,* Vol. IV, No. 1, Jan. 1956, p. 99. Alastair Reid has pointed out that having a sense of identity is having "good faith."

50[b] Cf. Kurt Lewin, "Intention, Will and Need," in David Rapaport, *Organization and Pathology of Thought,* Columbia University Press, 1951, p. 138.

50[c] Cf. Isenberg, "Natural Pride and Natural Shame," pp. 19-20.

50[d] Cf. pp. 150-2 on anxiety.

51[a] Piers and Singer, *Shame and Guilt,* pp. 11, 14, 16. This is in contrast to Fromm, who uses "guilt" to denote a failure to reach one's own ideals. See also p. 21 n. *c* above.

51[b] Plato, *The Symposium.*

51[c] *Othello,* IV, ii, 53-5.

52[a] *Ibid.,* 57-60.

52[b] Dmitri Furmanov, *Chapaev,* Moscow, 1934, p. 124, quoted in Rufus Mathewson, "The Hero in Soviet Literature" (manuscript), p. 323.

52[c] Ward Moore, *Bring the Jubilee,* Farrar, Straus, and Young, 1952, pp. 15-16.

53[a] Samuel A. Stouffer and Associates, *The American Soldier: Combat and Its Aftermath,* Princeton University Press, 1949, Vol. II, pp. 131-2. Cf. *ibid.,* pp. 196 ff. on teaching soldiers to accept fear in combat as normal. One thing apparent from this and similar studies is that shame can be somewhat eased if it is shared and if one can be assured that what one feels is perfectly natural under the circumstances.

53[b] Virginia Woolf, "The New Dress," in *A Haunted House and Other Short Stories,* Harcourt, Brace, 1944, pp. 47, 50, 55.

54[a] Genesis 9:21 and 23.

54[b] *King Lear,* IV, ii, 32-6.

54[c] Herman Melville, *Pierre, or the Ambiguities,* Dutton, 1929, p. 121.

54[d] *The Eternal Husband,* p. 384.

55[a] *Chance,* pp. 147, 192.

55[b] *Anna Karenina,* p. 12.

55[c] Jane Austen, *Pride and Prejudice,* Nelson, pp. 89-91.

55[d] Quoted in Aileen Pippett, *The Moth and the Star,* p. 26.

55[e] *Ibid.,* p. 14.

55[f] This attitude of immigrant children toward their parents has been described many times. See, for example, Everett V. Stonequist, *The Marginal Man,* Scribner's, 1937; Oscar Handlin, *The Uprooted: The Epic Story of the Great Migrations that Made the American People,* Little, Brown, 1951.

56[a] "The person who can witness another person's humiliation is said in our society to be 'heartless' just as he who can unfeelingly participate in his own defacement is thought to be 'shameless.'" (Erving Goffman, "On Face-Work," p. 215.)

57[a] St. Augustine, *Confessions,* trans. by J. G. Pilkington, in *A Select Library of the Nicene and Post-Nicene Fathers,* Christian Literature Company, 1886, Vol. I, Book VII, Chaps. 10, 11.

58[a] *Emmy Lou,* pp. 144-8.

59[a] *Of Human Bondage,* pp. 58-61.

59[b] *Middlemarch,* Chatto and Windus, Zodiac Press, 1950, pp. 196, 204-05.

59[c] *Anna Karenina,* pp. 374-5.

60[a] Harold D. Lasswell, among others, has described the particularly confusing, and at the same time particularly coercive, standards that middle-class parents, implicitly or explicitly, set for their children. (*Power and Personality,* Norton, 1948, pp. 47-9 and throughout.)

61[a] II Samuel 18:33. Cf. the statement of Admetos

> Men who never marry, men who have no children,
> Each of them has one life to live: his own;
> And a man can endure the pain of a single life.

(Euripides, *Alcestis,* an English version by Dudley Fitts and Robert Fitzgerald, Harcourt, Brace, 1936, Scene IV, Kommos.)

63[a] Handlin, *The Uprooted,* pp. 240, 243-4.

63[b] *Ibid.,* p. 108.

63[c] Thomas Hardy, *The Return of the Native,* Macmillan, 1922, p. 475.

63[d] *King Lear,* IV, i, 36-7.

64[a] See George Eliot's account of Bulstrode, *Middlemarch,* pp. 586-7.

65[a] *Chance,* p. 221.

65[b] Nancy Wilson Ross, *The Left Hand Is the Dreamer,* William Sloane, 1947, p. 196.

65[c] Robert K. Merton, "Social Structure and Anomie," in *Social Theory and Social Structure,* Free Press, 1949, pp. 125-49, especially pp. 128, 146, 149.

65[d] It is notable that the only full-length study of daydreams is Varendonck's published in 1921 (J. Varendonck, *The Psychology of Daydreams,* Allen and Unwin, 1921). Cf. Ernst Kris, *Psychoanalytic Explorations in Art,* International Universities Press, 1952, pp. 310-11 and 314-15.

66[a] *The Scartlet Letter,* p. 101.

66[b] Cf. Piers and Singer, *Shame and Guilt,* pp. 20-1.

66[c] See, for example, such confession of crimes one has not committed, after the mental torture of concentration camps, cited in William Sargant, *Battle for the Mind,* Chap. IX.

66[d] Rebecca West, "There Is No Conversation," in *The Harsh Voice,* Doubleday, Doran, 1935, p. 67.

67[a] Carson McCullers, *The Member of the Wedding,* Houghton Mifflin, 1946, p. 141.

67[b] Piers and Singer, *Shame and Guilt,* pp. 11, 16.

68[a] John Donne, *Complete Poetry and Selected Prose,* ed. by John Hayward, Random House, 1930, p. 513.

68[b] See Kurt Goldstein, "The Effect Of Brain Damage On The Personality," pp. 256-7; see also his *The Organism: A Holistic Approach to Biology Derived from Pathological Data in Man,* American Book Co., 1939, pp. 195-7, 292-5, and *Human Nature in the Light of Psychopathology,* Harvard University Press, 1940, pp. 109, 140-2. Cf. Freud's association of certain psychotic states with fears of annihilation. (Ruth Munroe, *Schools of Psychoanalytic Thought,* Dryden Press, 1955, pp. 288-9.)

68[c] *Autobiography of a Schizophrenic Girl,* with Analytic Interpretation by Marguerite Sechehaye, Grune and Stratton, 1951, pp. 4, 5.

69[a] R. G. Collingwood, *An Autobiography,* Oxford University Press, 1939, pp. 4-5.

69[b] Karl Marx and Friedrich Engels, *The German Ideology,* Parts I and II, International Publishers Company, 1939, pp. 74-5; Marx, "Alienated Labor," Three Essays Selected from the *Economic Philosophical Manuscripts,* mimeographed, trans. by Rita Stone.

69[c] See Edith Weigert, "Existentialism and Its Relations to Psychotherapy," *Psychiatry,* Vol. 12, No. 4, Nov. 1949, pp. 399-412.

69[d] Freud, *The Problem of Anxiety,* Psychoanalytic Quarterly Press and Norton, 1936, pp. 67-8 and throughout.

69[e] Ruth Munroe believes that Fromm overstresses the fear of being alone and insignificant until it becomes a kind of primary drive like Horney's need for security and Adler's need for superiority. (*Schools of Psychoanalytic Thought,* p. 397.) An outcome of this is what she regards as his overemphasis on the emptiness of the marketing orientation which, in her view, describes the era of Kafka and Ibsen rather than the present. (*Ibid.,* p. 476.)

70[a] *The Member of the Wedding,* p. 28. See also Carson McCullers, *The Heart Is a Lonely Hunter,* Houghton Mifflin, 1940, p. 257.

70[b] Elizabeth Bowen, *The Death of the Heart,* Knopf, 1939, p. 133.

70[c] Stephen Spender, *World Within World,* Harcourt, Brace, 1951, p. 141.

70[d] Virginia Woolf, *Night and Day,* Harcourt, Brace, 1920, pp. 274-5.

70[e] Kafka, *The Trial,* p. 75.

71[a] V. S. Pritchett, review of Guy de Maupassant, *A Woman's Life, New Statesman and Nation,* December 3, 1949.

71[b] V. S. Pritchett, "The Cat's Eye View," *New Statesman and Nation,* June 4, 1955. Pritchett also says that this is not the whole of de Maupassant.

75[a] See, for example, A. H. Maslow, *Motivation and Personality,* Harper, 1954, p. xi and Chap. XI.

75[b] Lancelot L. Whyte, *The Next Development in Man,* Holt, 1948, p. 67.

76[a] David Hume, *Treatise on Human Nature,* Everyman ed., Vol. I, pp. 238-40.

76[b] Cf. Solomon E. Asch, *Social Psychology,* Prentice-Hall, 1952, p. 280.

76[c] See Gilbert Ryle, Introduction, in A. J. Ayer and others, *The Revolution in Philosophy,* Macmillan, 1956, pp. 6, 7. Gottlob Frege and F. H. Bradley distinguished psychology sharply from logic and philosophy.

77[a] William Graham Sumner, *Folkways,* Ginn and Company, 1906, p. 3.

78[a] John W. M. Whiting and Irwin L. Child, *Child Training and Personality: A Cross-Cultural Study,* Yale University Press, 1953, pp. 8, 9, 10, 16, 117, 35; also pp. 50-4.

78[b] Parsons and Shils, *Toward a General Theory of Action,* pp. 6, 476, 481-3.

78[c] Robert R. Sears, "Social Behavior and Personality Development," in Parsons and Shils, *Toward a General Theory of Action,* p. 476.

78[d] Parsons and Shils, *Toward a General Theory of Action,* p. 6.

78[e] Sears, "Social Behavior and Personality Development," p. 476.

79[a] Parsons, *The Social System,* p. 481.

79[b] *Ibid.,* p. 201.

79[c] Sears, "Social Behavior and Personality Development," p. 472.

79[d] Parsons, *The Social System,* p. 133.

79[e] *Ibid.,* p. 535. Cf. Parsons and Shils' statement that equilibrium can be moving, not static. (*Toward a General Theory of Action,* p. 107.)

79[f] Parsons and Shils, *Toward a General Theory of Action,* p. 6.

80[a] See Ludwig von Bertalanffy, *Problems of Life: An Evaluation of Modern Biological Thought,* Watts and Co., 2d ed., 1952.

80[b] Edward C. Tolman, "A Psychological Model," in Parsons and Shils, *Toward a General Theory of Action,* p. 319. "Intervening variables" are said by the persons who use this term to be directly derived from the empirical data and to be required by the data as principles of explanation, whereas "hypothetical constructs" are more independent productions not so directly derived from the data. There may be something to be said for the view that one man's intervening variable is another man's hypothetical construct. It all depends upon what, in view of one's training and postulates, one believes can be directly derived from empirical data as a necessary principle of explanation.

80[c] Else Frenkel-Brunswick; "Personality Theory and Perception," in Robert R. Blake and Glenn V. Ramsey, eds., *Perception: An Approach to Personality,* Ronald Press, 1951, p. 356.

80[d] Dorothy Lee, "Lineal and Nonlineal Codifications of Reality," *Psychosomatic Medicine,* Vol. 12, No. 2, May 1950, pp. 91-2.

81[a] *Ibid.,* pp. 90, 91, 92, 97.

81[b] Dorothy Lee, "Linguistic Reflection of Wintu Thought," *International Journal of American Linguistics,* Vol. X, No. 4, Oct. 1944, pp. 181 and 185, and "Notes on the Conception of Self Among the Wintu Indians," *Journal of Abnormal and Social Psychology,* Vol. 45, No. 3, July 1950. Gordon Allport, Henry A. Murray, Kurt Lewin, Kurt Goldstein, and others raise similar questions about this kind of cause and effect, this part-to-whole sequence which will be discussed later.

81[c] Anna Freud, *The Ego and the Mechanisms of Defence,* International Universities Press, 1946, p. 30.

82[a] Anna Freud says: "All through childhood a maturation process is at work which . . . aims at perfecting [ego] functions, at rendering them more and more objective and *independent of the emotions* until they can become as accurate and reliable as a mechanical apparatus." ("Indication for Child Analysis," *Psychoanalytic Study of the Child,* Vol. I, 1945, p. 144. Italics mine.) Adelaide McF. Johnson comments on Anna Freud's view of the ego as a separate entity: "Is . . . not [Anna Freud's phrase 'the human ego by its very nature'] the logical error of petitio principii . . . in which a definition which has not been proved is smuggled into the sequence of an argument? 'By its very nature . . .' is an arbitrary postulation of what remains to be proved. Apparently Anna Freud assumed that the something within the ego itself, independent of outside influences and parental attitudes (and presumably, independent of heredity), is operating." ("Some Etiological Aspects of Repression, Guilt, and Hostility," *Psychoanalytic Quarterly*, Vol. XX, No. 4, Oct. 1951, p. 513.)

Erikson points out that the view that the ego can become independent of the emotions and like a mechanical apparatus reflects the mechanistic concepts of cause and effect of an earlier science. (Erikson, "Ego Development and Historical Change," p. 390.)

82[b] Sears, "Social Behavior and Personality Development," p. 468.

82[c] Whiting and Child, *Child Training and Personality*, p. 1.

82[d] "Culture and Personality," say Kluckhohn and Murray, "is as lopsided as biology and personality." (*Personality in Nature, Society and Culture*, pp. 62-3.)

82[e] Ernest Jones, *Sigmund Freud*, Hogarth Press, Vol. II, 1955, pp. 356-8.

82[f] Melvin H. Marx, ed., *Psychological Theory: Contemporary Readings*, Macmillan, 1951, p. 13.

83[a] See, for example, Freud, "The Predisposition to Obsessional Neurosis" (1913), *Collected Papers*, Vol. II, p. 128; Parsons and Shils, *Toward a General Theory of Action*, pp. 5, 9; Frenkel-Brunswick, "Personality Theory and Perception," p. 359; John Dollard and Neal E. Miller, *Personality and Psychotherapy: An Analysis in Terms of Learning, Thinking, and Culture*, McGraw-Hill, 1950, p. 103.

83[b] Jones, *Sigmund Freud*, Vol. I, 1953, p. 46.

83[c] *Ibid.*, pp. 236, 329, 381.

84[a] *Ibid.*, pp. 269, 402-3, 405, 410, 420.

84[b] Erikson, "The First Psychoanalyst," *The Yale Review*, Vol. XLVI, No. 1, Sept. 1956, p. 40.

84[c] See von Bertalanffy, "Some Considerations on Growth in Its Physical and Mental Aspects," *The Merrill-Palmer Quarterly*, Vol. III, No. 1, Fall 1956.

84[d] Erikson, "Freud's 'The Origins of Psychoanalysis,'" *The International Journal of Psychoanalysis*, Vol. XXXVI, Part I, 1951, p. 7.

84[e] Freud, *Three Contributions to the Theory of Sex* in *Basic Writings*, p. 611. Cf. also "Certain Neurotic Mechanisms in Jealousy, Paranoia and Homosexuality," (1922), *Collected Papers*, Vol. II, pp. 238-9.

85[a] "On Narcissism," p. 33. Cf. also p. 55.

85[b] *Ibid.*, pp. 45, 57; also pp. 46-7.

85[c] "Certain Neurotic Mechanisms in Jealousy, Paranoia and Homosexuality," p. 239.

85[d] Freud, *A General Introduction to Psychoanalysis*, Liveright, 1935, p. 243.

85[e] Freud, *An Outline of Psychoanalysis*, Norton, 1949, p. 32.

85[f] Therese Benedek, "Personality Development," in Franz Alexander and Helen Ross, eds., *Dynamic Psychiatry*, University of Chicago Press, 1952, p. 74.

85[g] *Ibid.*, p. 107

86[a] Rapaport, "On the Psycho-analytic Theory of Thinking," *International Journal of Psychoanalysis,* Vol. XXI, Part III, 1950, p. 6. See also his *Organization and Pathology of Thought,* Part VII.

86[b] Glenn Negley, "Cybernetics and Theories of Mind," *Journal of Philosophy,* Vol. XLVIII, No. 19, Sept. 13, 1951, pp. 577-81.

87[a] *Middlemarch,* p. 84.

87[b] E. M. Forster, *A Passage to India,* Harcourt, Brace, 1924, p. 254.

88[a] See, for example, Dollard and Miller, *Personality and Psychotherapy,* especially pp. 13, 120, 124, 377.

88[b] Munroe, *Schools of Psychoanalytic Thought,* p. 95. "Conflict-free" is used in both a wide and a narrow sense. In a narrow sense it may mean freedom from such conflicts as interfere with at least minimal functioning. In a wider sense it may imply that it is desirable for a person to live with the least conflict possible, in contrast to Goldstein's view that ability to live with conflict is necessary for the healthy, creative person.

89[a] See Munroe, *Schools of Psychoanalytic Thought,* pp. 111-12; also pp. 229, 617-19, and 642, for her discussion of drives and subsystems. Most analysts, she believes, actually mean compensation when they talk of sublimation. Munroe uses the term "drive system" to emphasize the inseparability of inner needs and direction toward goals. (*Ibid.*, p. 112.)

89[b] *Ibid.*, pp. 68, 111; cf. also p. 229.

89[c] Andras Angyal, *Foundations for a Science of Personality,* The Commonwealth Fund, 1941, p. 268. Angyal uses the term "biospheric constellation."

89[d] See Schachtel, "The Development of Focal Attention and the Emergence of Reality," pp. 317, 321-2.

90[a] *Three Contributions to the Theory of Sex,* p. 593.

90[b] "The Dynamics of the Transference" (1912), *Collected Papers,* Vol. II, p. 319.

90[c] "Analysis Terminable and Interminable" (1937), *Collected Papers,* Vol. V, p. 330.

90[d] *An Outline of Psychoanalysis,* p. 19.

90[e] *Ibid.*, p. 22.

90[f] "On The Transformation Of Instincts With Special Reference to Anal Eroticism" (1916), *Collected Papers,* Vol. II, p. 166.

90[g] *An Outline of Psychoanalysis,* p. 24.

90[h] "On Narcissism," p. 49. In this important paper Freud appears to be struggling with, at the same time that he reasserts, his compensatory theory. For example, he takes issue with Adler and asserts that excellent achievement may spring from superior as well as inferior organic endowment. (*Ibid.*, p. 56.)

90[i] Freud, *Civilization and Its Discontents,* Jonathan Cape & Harrison Smith, 1930, p. 87.

91[a] Freud, *Group Psychology and the Analysis of the Ego,* International Psycho-analytic Press, 1922, p. 54.

91[b] *Ibid.,* p. 88.

91[c] *Ibid.,* pp. 1, 2.

91[d] " 'Civilized' Sexual Morality and Modern Nervousness" (1908), *Collected Papers,* Vol. II, p. 82.

91[e] *Civilization and Its Discontents,* p. 123.

91[f] *Ibid.,* p. 63.

91[g] *Group Psychology and the Analysis of the Ego,* p. 10.

91[h] "The Predisposition to Obsessional Neurosis" (1913), *Collected Papers,* Vol. II, pp. 130-1; cf. p. 128.

92[a] "Negation" (1925), *Collected Papers,* Vol. V, p. 184.

92[b] "On Narcissism," p. 51.

92[c] Benedek, "Personality Development," pp. 107, 105, 90.

92[d] Melanie Klein and Joan Riviere, *Love, Hate, and Repressions,* Hogarth Press, 1937, p. 107.

92[e] See *e.g.,* Heinz Hartmann, "Ego Psychology and the Problem of Adaptation," in Rapaport, *Organization and Pathology of Thought,* pp. 380, 370; Heinz Hartmann, Ernst Kris, Rudolph M. Loewenstein, "Comments on the Formation of Psychic Structure," in *The Psychoanalytic Study of the Child,* Vol. II, 1946, pp. 11-37.

92[f] Heinz Hartmann, "Mutual Influences in the Development of the Ego and the Id," *The Psychoanalytic Study of the Child,* Vol. VII, 1952, p. 15. Cf. Hartmann, "On Rational and Irrational Action," in Geza Roheim, ed., *Psychoanalysis and the Social Sciences,* International Universities Press, 1947, Vol. I, pp. 363-4, and "The Psychoanalytic Theory of the Ego," in *The Psychoanalytic Study of the Child,* Vol. V, 1950, pp. 74-96.

93[a] David Rapaport, "Paul Schilder's Contribution to the Theory of Thought-Processes," *International Journal of Psycho-analysis,* Vol. XXXII, Part IV, 1951, p. 5. Rapaport says, however, that Schilder, unlike Horney and Fromm, always kept "primary drives" in mind.

93[b] *Ibid.,* pp. 7, 8. "Object" is used by Schilder more widely than in the limited Freudian sense.

93[c] David Rapaport, *The Organization and Pathology of Thought,* pp. 690, 702.

93[d] *Ibid.,* p. 720.

94[a] See, for example, *ibid.,* pp. 691, 694.

94[b] Cf. George Meredith, *An Essay on Comedy* and Henri Bergson, *Laughter,* Doubleday Anchor Books, 1956. Cf. also Orrin E. Klapp, "The Fool as a Social Type," *The American Journal of Sociology,* Vol. 55, No. 2, Sept. 1949, pp. 157-62.

94[c] Thomas Hobbes, *Leviathan,* Cambridge University Press, 1904, Part

I, Chap. VI, p. 34. Cf. Freud, *Wit and Its Relation to the Unconscious,* in *Basic Writings.*

95[a] Ernst Kris, *Psychoanalytic Explorations in Art,* International Universities Press, 1952, p. 208.

95[b] *Ibid.,* p. 220.

95[c] *Ibid.,* p. 175.

95[d] *Ibid.,* p. 188.

95[e] *Ibid.,* pp. 232-3.

95[f] *Ibid.,* p. 216.

95[g] *Ibid.,* pp. 208-10; see also pp. 181-3.

95[h] Morris W. Brody, "The Meaning of Laughter," *Psychoanalytic Quarterly,* Vol. XIX, No. 2, Apr. 1950, p. 201.

96[a] Sidney Tarachow, "Remarks on the Comic Process and Beauty," *Psychoanalytic Quarterly,* Vol. XVIII, No. 2, Apr. 1949, pp. 224-5.

96[b] Bertram D. Lewin, *The Psychoanalysis of Elation,* Norton, 1950, p. 91.

96[c] Edith Jacobson, "The Child's Laughter," *The Psychoanalytic Study of the Child,* Vol. II, 1946, p. 46.

96[d] *King Lear,* III, i, 16, 17.

97[a] *The Organism,* p. 333.

97[b] *Toward a General Theory of Action,* pp. 18-19.

97[c] *Personality and Psychotherapy,* pp. 3, 4, 130, 135.

97[d] *Child Training and Personality,* p. 45.

97[e] "Social Behavior and Personality Development," p. 477.

97[f] Georg Simmel, *Conflict,* trans. by Kurt H. Wolff, The Free Press, 1955, quoted in Lewis A. Coser, *The Functions of Social Conflict,* The Free Press, 1956, pp. 60, 91.

97[g] Lasswell, *Power and Personality,* p. 49. Lasswell is speaking here particularly of the middle class.

98[a] Harold D. Lasswell, *World Politics and Personal Insecurity,* McGraw-Hill, 1935, p. 73.

98[b] "A Psychological Model," p. 332.

98[c] Dorothy Lee, "Are Basic Needs Ultimate?" *Journal of Abnormal and Social Psychology,* Vol. 43, No. 3, July 1948, p. 392.

99[a] Kluckhohn and Murray, *Personality in Nature, Society, and Culture,* p. 43.

99[b] "Formulations Regarding the Two Principles in Mental Functioning" (1911), *Collected Papers,* Vol. IV.

99[c] *Ibid.,* p. 18. Cf. also Freud, *Beyond the Pleasure Principle,* Hogarth Press and Institute of Psycho-analysis, 1948.

99[d] "On Rational and Irrational Action," p. 383.

100[a] "Ego Psychology and the Problem of Adaptation," pp. 381 and 382, n. 62. Cf. William James (*The Principles of Psychology,* Holt, 1890, Vol. II, pp. 549 ff.) for another statement of the pleasure principle.

100[b] "Fragment of an Analysis of a Case of Hysteria" (1905), *Collected Papers,* Vol. III, pp. 37-8.

100[c] "Mourning and Melancholia" (1917), *Collected Papers,* Vol. IV, pp. 154, 166.

101[a] *Ibid.,* p. 159.

101[b] *Civilization and Its Discontents,* pp. 57-8.

101[c] *Ibid.,* p. 27. Cf. *Three Contributions to the Theory of Sex,* pp. 620-31.

101[d] *Civilization and Its Discontents,* p. 29.

101[e] *Ibid.,* pp. 25, 33, 35.

101[f] Proust, *The Captive,* Modern Library, p. 291.

102[a] Paul Federn, *Ego Psychology and the Psychoses,* Basic Books, 1952, p. 262.

102[b] Whiting and Child, *Child Training and Personality,* p. 18.

102[c] *Toward a General Theory of Action,* p. 5.

102[d] Whiting and Child, *Child Training and Personality,* p. 29; see also pp. 50-4.

103[a] *Personality and Psychotherapy,* p. 9.

103[b] *Ibid.,* p. 42, n. 15.

103[c] *Ibid.,* p. 45; cf. p. 47.

103[d] *Ibid.,* p. 427.

103[e] O. H. Mowrer, "Stimulus-Response Theory of Anxiety," in M. H. Marx, *Psychological Theory,* p. 495.

103[f] Harold D. Lasswell, "Person, Personality, Group, Culture," in Patrick Mullahy, *A Study of Interpersonal Relations,* pp. 318-19.

Talcott Parsons discusses "particularism" in relations between persons, and this may refer to mutual love; I am not entirely sure of his meaning. When he speaks of "specifically delimited instrumental obligation" he would seem to exclude mutuality; when he speaks of "pursuit of a segregated specific interest" or "expectation of specific effective expression" he may include mutuality. (*The Social System,* pp. 86, 104.) Lasswell's description of "indulgence" as increase of "deference, income, and safety" would seem definitely to exclude mutual love between persons.

104[a] Lasswell, *Power and Personality,* p. 126.

104[b] See Chap. V, pp. 186-91 for discussion of social roles.

104[c] Hermann Rorschach, *Psychodiagnostics,* Verlag Hans Huber, 1942, p. 94 and throughout.

104[d] Dollard and Miller, *Personality and Psychotherapy,* p. 4.

105[a] *Ibid.,* p. 36.

105[b] *Ibid.,* p. 123.

105[c] *Ibid.,* pp. 292-3.

106[a] John Stuart Mill, "Bentham," in F. R. Leavis, *Mill on Bentham and Coleridge,* Chatto and Windus, 1950, pp. 63, 59, 61-3, 66.

106[b] *Ibid.,* pp. 66-8.

107[a] Cf. Henry A. Murray's statement that "Instantaneous records . . . or observations regulated by the clock are incongruent with reality." ("Toward a Classification of Interactions," p. 437.)

109[a] Sidney Hook, "On Historical Understanding" review of Karl R. Popper, *The Open Society and Its Enemies,* Princeton University Press, 1950, *Partisan Review,* Vol. XV, No. 2, Feb. 1948, p. 231.

109[b] *The Social System,* p. 486.

109[c] Coser, *The Functions of Social Conflict,* p. 23; see also pp. 26-7, 34. Coser approaches Parsons' position when he describes the ways in which social conflict can contribute to the maintenance of social structures (pp. 151 ff.).

110[a] "Are Basic Needs Ultimate?" pp. 392-3.

110[b] See, for example, "Ego Psychology and the Problem of Adaptation," p. 377 n., and "Psychoanalysis and the Concept of Health," *International Journal of Psychoanalysis,* Vol. 20, 1939, Parts III and IV, pp. 308-21.

110[c] *Organization and Pathology of Thought,* pp. 689-91 and throughout.

110[d] Norbert Wiener, *Cybernetics,* John Wiley and Sons, 1948, p. 53.

111[a] *Ibid.*

111[b] Kenneth W. Spence, "Types of Constructs in Psychology," in M. H. Marx, *Psychological Theory,* p. 77.

111[c] *World Politics and Personal Insecurity,* pp. 4-5.

111[d] Cf. Kingsley Davis, "Mental Hygiene and the Class Structure," in Patrick Mullahy, *A Study of Interpersonal Relations,* especially pp. 373-85.

111[e] Norman Reider, "The Concept of Normality," *Psychoanalytic Quarterly,* Vol. XIX, No. 1, Jan. 1950, p. 43. See also Helen M. Lynd, "Must Psychology Aid Reaction?" *The Nation,* Jan. 15, 1949.

111[f] Cf. Marc Bloch, *The Historian's Craft,* trans. by Peter Putnam, Knopf, 1953, especially pp. 27-8, and Chap. IV. Cf. also Collingwood, *An Autobiography,* pp. 101-06.

112[a] Paul A. Baran, *The Political Economy of Growth,* Monthly Review Press, 1957.

112[b] Thomas I. Cook, review of Harold D. Lasswell and Abraham Kaplan, *Power and Society: A Framework for Political Inquiry,* Yale University Press, 1950, the *Journal of Philosophy,* Vol. XLVIII, No. 22, Oct. 25, 1951, pp. 697-8.

113[a] See Helen M. Lynd, "The Nature of Historical Objectivity," *Journal of Philosophy,* Vol. XLVII, No. 2, Jan. 19, 1950. Cf. Gunnar Myrdal's discussion of the concealed values of American social scientists who study the American Negro and the effect of these values on their selection and formulation of problems, in *An American Dilemma,* Harper, 1944.

113[b] Barker Fairley, *A Study of Goethe,* Oxford, Clarendon Press, 1947, pp. 231-2.

113[c] "The First Psychoanalyst," p. 42.

113[d] Cf. Maurice Mandelbaum, *The Problem of Historical Knowledge,* Liveright, 1938, pp. 203-04.

114[a] M. H. Marx, *Psychological Theory,* p. 9.

115[a] *Ibid.,* p. 11.

115[b] David C. McClelland, *Personality,* Dryden Press, 1951, p. 279.

115[c] Quoted in McClelland, *Personality,* p. 275.

115[d] *Schools of Psychoanalytical Thought,* pp. 229, 616.

115[e] *Ibid.,* p. 273.

115[f] *Ibid.,* p. 228.

115[g] *Ibid.,* p. 165.

115[h] *Ibid.,* p. 459.

115[i] *Ibid.,* p. 155.

115[j] *Ibid.,* p. 241.

115[k] *Ibid.,* p. 273.

115[l] See also *ibid.,* pp. 90, 181, 272, 329, 364, 567 for Munroe's emphasis on the multidimensional character of Freud's theory.

115[m] *Ibid.,* pp. 94 and 109.

115[n] *Ibid.,* p. 239 n.

116[a] *Ibid.,* p. 94.

116[b] "The Development of Focal Attention and the Emergence of Reality," p. 318.

116[c] *Ibid.,* p. 324.

117[a] *Ibid.*

117[b] Lionel Trilling, *The Liberal Imagination: Essays on Literature and Society,* Viking, 1951, pp. 48, 52, 57.

117[c] *Eros and Civilization.* Marcuse in *Reason and Revolution* (Oxford University Press, 1941) makes clear his analysis of Hegel and Marx that is implied in *Eros and Civilization.*

118[a] D. F. Pears, "Logical Atomism," in Ayer, *The Revolution in Philosophy,* pp. 52-3. Cf., however, Ryle's statement that the goal of the positivists of the Vienna Circle was no longer to isolate simple namables but to isolate simple statables; the sentence, not the part of speech, became the unit. (Introduction, in *ibid.,* p. 10.) See, for example, Charles W. Morris, *Signs, Language, and Behavior,* Prentice-Hall, 1946; A. J. Ayer, *Language, Truth, and Logic,* Gollancz, 1947.

118[b] Morris, *Signs, Language, and Behavior,* pp. 212-13.

118[c] Joost A. M. Meerloo, *Conversation and Communication: A Psychological Inquiry Into Language and Human Relations,* International Universities Press, 1952, p. 87.

118[d] See Erikson, "On the Sense of Inner Identity," p. 354.

119[a] George Herbert Mead calls these signs "significant symbols." It is through the use of such words of fixed meaning, he believes, that one can put oneself into the position of the hearer, "the particular other," and can answer questions to oneself as to another, "the generalized other." (George Herbert Mead, *Mind, Self, & Society,* University of Chicago Press, 1934.) See also Hans Garth and C. Wright Mills, *Character and Social Structure,* Harcourt, Brace, 1953.

119[b] Ernst Cassirer, *An Essay on Man: An Introduction to a Philosophy of Human Culture,* Yale University Press, 1944, p. 32.

120[a] "Personality Development," p. 74.

120[b] Lawrence S. Kubie, "Body Symbolism and Language," *Psychoanalytic Quarterly,* Vol. III, No. 3, July 1934, pp. 430-44.

120[c] Dollard and Miller, *Personality and Psychotheraphy,* pp. 99-100.

120[d] Robert H. Thouless, "The Affective Function of Language," in Reymert, *Feelings and Emotions,* p. 509.

120[e] "A Psychological Model," p. 332.

121[a] Emery Neff, *The Poetry of History,* Columbia University Press, 1947, pp. 31-2.

123[a] "Paul Schilder's Contribution to the Theory of Thought Processes," p. 1.

123[b] *Ibid.,* p. 9.

124[a] See, for example, "On Narcissism," p. 34.

124[b] Cf. von Bertalanffy, *Problems of Life,* pp. 149-50.

124[c] *Psychological Theory,* pp. 15-16.

125[a] See, for example, S. S. Stevens, "Psychology and the Science of Science," in M. H. Marx, *Psychological Theory,* pp. 21-54, and Alexander Koyré, "Influence of Philosophic Trends on the Formulation of Scientific Theories," *The Scientific Monthly,* Vol. 60, No. 2, Feb. 1955, pp. 107-11.

125[b] See Gregory Bateson, "Some Experiments in Thinking about Ethnographical Data," *Philosophy of Science,* Vol. 8, No. 1, Jan. 1941.

127[a] See von Bertalanffy, *Problems of Life,* pp. 12-14; Erwin Schroedinger, *What Is Life?,* Doubleday, 1956; George Gaylord Simpson, *The Meaning of Evolution,* Yale University Press, 1950; Kurt Goldstein, *The Organism* and *Human Nature in the Light of Psychopathology.*

127[b] Kurt Lewin, *A Dynamic Theory of Personality,* McGraw-Hill, 1935. Gardner Murphy and others use field theory as practically synonymous with holism. See Gardner Murphy, "Approaches to Personality," in M. H. Marx, *Psychological Theory,* pp. 522-5, and his *Personality: A Biosocial Approach to Origins and Structure,* Harper, 1947.

127[c] Heinz Hartmann, Ernst Kris, Rudolph M. Loewenstein, "Notes on the Theory of Aggression," in *The Psychoanalytic Study of the Child,* Vols. III-IV, International Universities Press, 1949, p. 13.

127[d] Urie Bronfenbrenner, "Toward an Integrated Theory of Personality," in Blake and Ramsey, *Perception: An Approach to Personality,* p. 209.

127[e] Littman and Rosen point out seven different meanings for the term molar and question the current usefulness of the molar-molecular distinction. (Richard A. Littman and Ephriam Rosen, "The Molar-Molecular Distinction," in M. H. Marx, *Psychological Theory*, pp. 144, 147-51.) M. H. Marx mentions three different types of field theory. (*Ibid.*, p. 298.)

128[a] Maslow, *Motivation and Personality*, p. 49.

129[a] Konrad Z. Lorenz, "The Role of Gestalt Perception," in Lancelot L. Whyte, *Aspects of Forms*, Lund Humphries, 1951, pp. 158-60.

129[b] See Max Wertheimer, *Productive Thinking*, Harper, 1945, and "Gestalt Theory," *Social Research*, Vol. XI, No. 1, Feb. 1944; Kurt Lewin, "The Nature of Field Theory," in M. H. Marx, *Psychological Theory*, and his *A Dynamic Theory of Personality*.

130[a] Henry A. Murray, "Toward a Classification of Interactions," in Parsons and Shils, *Toward a General Theory of Action*, p. 436. Cf. Murray's statement that ". . . trait psychology is over-concerned . . . with what is clearly manifested . . . with what is conscious, ordered and rational. It minimizes the importance of . . . irrational impulses and beliefs, infantile experiences, unconscious and inhibited drives. . . . Hence it does not seem fitted to cope with such phenomena as: dreams and fantasies, the behavior and thought of children or savages, neurotic symptoms . . . insanity and creative activity." (*Explorations in Personality*, Oxford University Press, 1938, p. 715.)

130[b] Paul Schilder, *Goals and Desires of Man: A Psychological Survey of Life*, Columbia University Press, 1942, p. 48.

130[c] Paul Schilder, *Mind: Perception and Thought in Their Constructive Aspects*, Columbia University Press, 1942, p. 305.

130[d] Paul Schilder, quoted in Rapaport, "Paul Schilder's Contribution to the Theory of Thought," p. 8.

130[e] *The Organism*, pp. 268-9. See also pp. 91 and 93.

131[a] *Ibid.*, p. 161

131[b] *Ibid.*, p. 271. See also Goldstein, "The Effect of Brain Damage on the Personality."

131[c] *Psychodiagnostics*, pp. 61-6 and throughout.

131[d] Ernest Schachtel, "The Dynamic Perception and the Symbolism of Form," *Psychiatry*, Vol. 4, No. 1, Feb. 1941; "On Color and Affect," *Psychiatry*, Vol. 6, No. 4, Nov. 1943; "Subjective Definitions of the Rorschach Test Situation and Their Effect on Test Performance," *Psychiatry*, Vol. 8, No. 4, Nov. 1945; "Projection and Its Relation to Character Attitudes and Creativity in the Kinesthetic Responses," *Psychiatry*, Vol. 13, No. 1, Feb. 1950; "The Development of Focal Attention and the Emergence of Reality."

131[e] "Dynamic Perception and the Symbolism of Form," pp. 79, 81, 91, 93, 79 n. 2.

132[a] *Schools of Psychoanalytic Thought*, p. 597.

132[b] *Ibid.*, p. 113.

134[a] See Jacob Loewenberg, Introduction to *Hegel: Selections*, Scribner's, 1929; Hegel, *The Phenomenology of Mind*, Swan Sonnenschein, 1910, especially Preface and Introduction, in Vol. I.

135[a] Lewin, *A Dynamic Theory of Personality*, Chap. I. Lewin is in this chapter inconsistent with his own multidimensional theory in advocating an antihistorical approach. His antihistorical view makes it difficult to understand how. time enters into his "continuous variation."

135[b] Hegel, *Phenomenology of Mind*, Vol. I, p. 27.

136[a] Some of these issues in physics are by no means finally settled. Max Planck regarded himself as in a minority among modern physicists in being a determinist, that is, in taking into account the full, concrete situation. But he also believed that this minority insisted on pushing questions farther than the majority and that these questions might sometime find answers. (*The Philosophy of Physics*, Norton, 1936, especially pp. 58, 65, 70-2, 82.) See also Philipp Frank, *Philosophy of Science: The Link Between Science and Philosophy*, Prentice-Hall, 1957.

P. W. Bridgman says that implied in the possibility of discovery beyond our present range "is the recognition that no element of a physical situation, no matter how apparently irrelevant or trivial, may be dismissed as without effect on the final result until proved to be without effect by actual experiment." (*The Logic of Modern Physics*, Macmillan, 1928, p. 3.)

In biology, too, evidence forces us to go beyond earlier and simpler concepts of causation. ". . . inheritance is not a mechanism where genes are connected machine-fashion with the visible characters they produce, but rather it is a flow of processes in which the genes interfere in definite ways." (Von Bertalanffy, *Problems of Life*, p. 73.)

136[b] *Interpretation of Dreams* in *Basic Writings*, p. 238, and "On Narcissism," p. 34.

136[c] Harry Stack Sullivan, *Conceptions of Modern Psychiatry*, William Alanson White Foundation, 1940, pp. 91, 100.

137[a] *The Image and Appearance of the Human Body*, pp. 217 and 203.

137[b] *Ibid.*, p. 179; and his *Goals and Desires of Man*, p. 124; *The Image and Appearance of the Human Body*, pp. 138-9.

137[c] *Mind: Perception and Thought*, pp. 180, 250.

138[a] *Goals and Desires of Man*, p. 212.

138[b] *The Organism*, pp. 80-1.

138[c] *Ibid.*, pp. 292, 4-5. Kurt R. Eissler questions this concurrent growth in awareness of sense of self and sense of objects. He thinks that this "correlated progress" is possible, but adds, "On the other hand, I could imagine that the child's gradual awareness of external reality preoccupies his mind to such an extent that a corresponding process regarding the child's own ego can set in only belatedly." ("Psychoanalytic Treatment of Delinquents," *Psychoanalytic Study of the Child,* Vol. V, 1950, pp. 111-12.)

138[d] *Psychodiagnostics,* p. 87 and throughout.

138[e] *Ibid.,* pp. 79, 82.

139[a] *Ibid.,* p. 38.

139[b] Wolfgang Köhler, *The Place of Value in a World of Facts,* Liveright, 1938, and Wertheimer, *Productive Thinking.*

139[c] Cf. also Blake and Ramsey, *Perception: An Approach to Personality.*

139[d] "The Dynamic Perception and the Symbolism of Form," p. 91.

139[e] "Projection and Its Relation to Character," p. 75.

139[f] *Ibid.,* p. 77, and "The Dynamic Perception and the Symbolism of Form," p. 95.

140[a] "The Development of Focal Attention and the Emergence of Reality," p. 310. Cf. Helen M. Lynd, "The Nature of Historical Objectivity."

140[b] T. S. Eliot, "The Metaphysical Poets," in *Selected Essays,* Faber and Faber, 1932, pp. 286-7.

140[c] Paraphrased from Eliot by F. O. Matthiessen, in *The Achievement of T. S. Eliot,* Oxford University Press, 1947, pp. 12-13.

141[a] Kurt Goldstein's term.

142[a] Cf. Piers and Singer, *Shame and Guilt,* pp. 11 and 16, and Lee, "Are Basic Needs Ultimate?"

142[b] Cf. Alexander, *Fundamentals of Psychoanalysis,* and Erikson, "The Problem of Ego Identity," p. 71.

142[c] Freud himself suggests some of these implications in "On Narcissism," p. 56.

143[a] "Toward a Classification of Interaction," p. 435.

143[b] "Emphasis on Molar Problems," in M. H. Marx, *Psychological Theory,* p. 166.

143[c] "Toward a Classification of Interaction," p. 443.

143[d] *Ibid.,* p. 445; see also p. 447.

143[e] *Ibid.,* p. 439. See also Allport, "Emphasis on Molar Problems," p. 163.

144[a] *Fundamentals of Psychoanalysis,* p. 43. Alexander explains that the discharge of erotic energy is one manifestation of the homeostatic principle. "Excess of unused energy disturbs homeostatic equilibrium and must therefore be discharged." (*Ibid.*)

George S. Klein makes the point that the concept of equilibrium is useful only if it is recognized that the kinds of balance and the means of reaching it are different for different people. ("The Personal World Through Perception," in Blake and Ramsey, *Perception: An Approach to Personality,* p. 330.)

144[b] *Goals and Desires of Man,* p. 220; cf. also p. 178.

144[c] *Image and Appearance of the Human Body,* p. 254.

144[d] *Goals and Desires of Man,* pp. 276-7.

145[a] Goldstein, *Human Nature in the Light of Psychopathology,* p. 111. Schilder criticizes Goldstein's account of amnesic aphasia as a disorder of categorical thinking. He believes that this is an oversimplified interpretation of the data. ("On the Development of Thoughts" in Rapaport, *Organization and Pathology of Thought,* pp. 564-5. See also *ibid.,* p. 567 n. 239 and p. 641 n. 149.)

145[b] *Human Nature in the Light of Psychopathology,* pp. 140-2.

145[c] *Schools of Psychoanalytic Thought,* pp. 111-12.

146[a] Radhakamal Mukerjee, *The Social Structure of Values,* Macmillan, 1949, pp. 156-7, 178-9, 180-1.

147[a] Boris Sidis, *The Psychology of Laughter,* Appleton, 1923, pp. 68-9, 70, 223. Sidis also recognizes that humor *may be* a compensation for weakness and aggression, a display of strength over weakness, and that the discomfiture of other people may be perceived as ludicrous, but, in his view, it is a distortion of humor to confine it to these situations. Jones dismisses Sidis as simply an intemperate disturber of Freudian theory. (*Sigmund Freud,* Vol. II, pp. 129-30.)

147[b] Henry A. Murray, "The Psychology of Humor," *Journal of Abnormal and Social Psychology,* Vol. 29, No. 1, Apr. 1934, p. 67.

147[c] Cf. Kenneth Burke, *Attitudes Toward History,* The New Republic Press, 1937, Vol. I, p. 121.

147[d] Quoted in Rufus Mathewson, "The Hero in Soviet Literature," p. 184.

147[e] Loewenberg, *Selections from Hegel,* p. xxi.

148[a] See, for example, Harry F. Harlow, "Mice, Monkeys, Men and Motives," *Psychological Review,* Vol. 60, No. 1, Jan. 1953, p. 25.

148[b] "Emphasis on Molar Problems," pp. 159, 161.

148[c] "Toward a Classification of Interaction," p. 450.

148[d] Edward C. Tolman, *Purposive Behavior in Animals and Men,* Century, 1932.

148[e] *Ibid.,* pp. 422-3. See also pp. 389-90 on intervening variables.

149[a] Harlow, "Mice, Monkeys, Men and Motives," pp. 23-9.

149[b] Cf. Ruth Munroe, *Schools of Psychoanalytic Thought,* p. 363.

149[c] "Are Basic Needs Ultimate?" pp. 393-4, 392.

150[a] *The Organism,* p. 86.

150[b] "The Effect of Brain Damage on the Personality," p. 251. David C. McClelland classes Goldstein's "monistic" theories of motivation with Freud's (*Personality,* p. 403). McClelland's classification calls attention to the necessity of recognizing subsystems between an over-all self-actualizing tendency and specific acts, but it misses the important distinction between the compensatory character of Freud's theory and the purposive character of Goldstein's theory of self-actualization.

150[c] Goldstein recognizes that there can be a degree of conflict and anxiety that is paralyzing, and he does not adopt the coping philosophy that tends to regard all reality as a threat. Jones speaks of the deep impression made on Freud by the phenomenon of conflict "which typically is between two opposing forces" (*Sigmund Freud,* Vol. II, p. 358), and contemporary Freudians such as Hartmann certainly do not minimize the importance of conflict in life. But the tendency is for Freudians to regard conflict as an unfortunate inevitability to be reduced for healthy living rather than as a possible source of increased individual strength and of historical development.

151[a] "The Anxiety-Neurosis" (1894), *Collected Papers,* Vol. I, pp. 97, 101.

151[b] Freud, *The Problem of Anxiety,* pp. 13, 75, 77 and throughout.

151[c] Harry Stack Sullivan, *The Meaning of Anxiety in Psychiatry and in Life,* William Alanson White Institute of Psychiatry, 1948, pp. 3, 4, 7.

151[d] "The Effect of Brain Damage on Personality," p. 257.

152[a] *The Organism,* p. 306. Cf. Hartmann's comment on individual differences in anxiety tolerance. ("Ego Psychology and the Problem of Adaptation," p. 385.)

152[b] *Human Nature in the Light of Psychopathology,* pp. 112-13.

153[a] As noted above, Marcuse attempts to translate Freud's psychological necessity into historical analysis, a criticism of capitalism and precapitalist societies; but I cannot find the basis for this in Freud. (Marcuse, *Eros and Civilization.*)

153[b] Freud, *Group Psychology and the Analysis of the Ego,* p. 78.

153[c] *Ibid.,* p. 54.

154[a] Lasswell's terms in "Person, Personality, Group, Culture," pp. 318-19 and *Power and Personality,* p. 126.

154[b] "Existentialism and Its Relation to Psychotherapy," pp. 403-04. Weigert uses Ludwig Binswanger's term the realm of Care for a situation dominated by power and anxiety. It is not entirely clear to what extent she takes into account the importance of a particular historical situation in shaping relations between persons and to what extent she thinks there can be modes of life independent of their historical setting.

155[a] *Goals and Desires of Man,* pp. 136-7.

155[b] *Ibid.,* p. 188.

156[a] Schachtel, "The Development of Focal Attention and the Emergence of Reality," p. 322.

156[b] *Psychodiagnostics,* p. 113.

156[c] *The Psychoanalysis of Elation,* p. 91 and throughout.

156[d] *Psychodiagnostics,* pp. 65, 71, 93, 104, and elsewhere.

157[a] See Sullivan, *Conceptions of Modern Psychiatry; The Meaning of Anxiety in Psychiatry and in Life; The Interpersonal Theory of*

Psychiatry, Norton, 1953; Patrick Mullahy, ed., *The Contributions of Harry Stack Sullivan*, Hermitage House, 1952.

157[b] Frieda Fromm-Reichmann, *Principles of Intensive Psychotherapy*, University of Chicago Press, 1950, and articles in *Psychiatry*.

157[c] Sechehaye, *Autobiography of a Schizophrenic Girl*.

157[d] *The Uprooted*, pp. 96-7.

158[a] Helen Mims, "The Communal Mind and the Master Artificer" (unpublished), especially Section IV, pp. 44-57.

158[b] "Greece," in Margaret Mead, ed., *Cultural Patterns and Technical Change*, Tensions and Technology Series, United Nations, 1953, pp. 77, 80.

158[c] Lee uses the modern Greek word for shame, *entrope*, meaning "modesty, decency, propriety, self-consciousness, embarrassment, turning inward." ("Greece," p. 81.) The classical Greek word for shame, *aidos*, is defined by H. D. F. Kitto as meaning "inner compulsion" (*The Greeks*, Penguin, 1951, p. 247), and by Zimmern as a "vague sense of respect for gods and men and shame of wrongdoing before earth and sky." (*The Greek Commonwealth*, Oxford University Press, 1922, p. 121.) As noted in Chap. I, *aischyne* was more related to man-made laws.

158[d] *The Greeks and the Irrational*, p. 34.

158[e] Cf. Helen Merrell Lynd, *England in the Eighteen-Eighties: Toward a Social Basis for Freedom*, Oxford University Press, 1945, especially Chaps. III, V, X, XI.

159[a] William H. Whyte, Jr., *The Organization Man*, Simon and Schuster, 1956.

159[b] Cf. Erikson, *Childhood and Society*, pp. 129-31; "Growth and Crises of the 'Healthy Personality,'" in Kluckhohn and Murray, *Personality in Nature, Society, and Culture*, pp. 221-2; "On the Sense of Inner Identity," p. 363.

160[a] Weigert, "Existentialism and Its Relation to Psychotherapy," pp. 404-05.

160[b] See Munroe, *Schools of Psychoanalytic Thought*, pp. 138-41 for discussion of Roheim's view of cultural concepts.

Munroe notes the impact of cultural findings upon psychoanalysts: that Karen Horney "almost alone among psychoanalysts" shows the effect of contradictory ideals in the culture upon the individual (*ibid.*, p. 386); that Fromm's chief contribution is his insistence on the principle of constant interactions between social trends and psychological trends (*ibid.*, pp. 396-7).

161[a] "Application of Psychoanalytic Concepts to Social Science," *Psychoanalytic Quarterly*, Vol. XIX, No. 3, July 1950, p. 387.

162[a] *Goals and Desires of Man*, pp. 178-9; see also p. 116, and *Mind: Perception and Thought*, p. 365.

162[b] Heinz Hartmann, Ernst Kris, and R. M. Loewenstein, "Some Psychoanalytic Comments on 'Culture and Personality,'" in G. B. Wilbur and W. Münsterberger, eds., *Psychoanalysis and Culture,* International Universities Press, 1951.

162[c] "The Problem of Ego Identity," pp. 107-08.

162[d] Abram Kardiner, *The Individual and His Society,* Columbia University Press, 1939; *The Psychological Frontiers of Society,* Columbia University Press, 1945; *Sex and Morality,* Bobbs-Merrill, 1954.

163[a] "The Dynamic Perception and the Symbolism of Form," p. 79 and throughout.

163[b] "The Development of Focal Attention and the Emergence of Reality."

163[c] *Ibid.,* pp. 309-10.

164[a] *Ibid.,* pp. 317-18. Cf. pp. 321-2 on the development of thought and focal attention only if there is relative freedom from pressure of needs and tensions.

164[b] Rudolf Arnheim, "The Gestalt Theory of Expression," *Psychological Review,* Vol. 56, No. 3, May 1949, p. 160. See also Arnheim's "Perceptual Abstraction and Art," *Psychological Review,* Vol. 54, No. 2, March 1947; and "A Review of Proportion," *The Journal of Aesthetics and Art Criticism,* Vol. XIV, No. 1, Sept. 1955.

164[c] Frederick J. Teggart, *The Theory of History,* Yale University Press, 1925, p. 157.

165[a] Collingwood, *An Autobiography,* p. 100. Cf. also Collingwood's statement: "Obscure provinces [of history] always rather appeal to me. Their obscurity is a challenge; you have to invent new methods for studying them, and then you will probably find that the cause of their obscurity is some defect in the methods hitherto used . . . In this sense knowledge advances by proceeding not 'from the known to the unknown,' but from the 'unknown' to the 'known.'" (*Ibid.,* p. 86.)

165[b] *The Social Sciences in Historical Study: A Report of the Committee on Historiography,* Social Science Research Council, 1954. See also *Theory and Practice in Historical Study,* published by the Social Science Research Council in 1946.

165[c] "National Character" in A. L. Kroeber, ed., *Anthropology Today,* University of Chicago Press, 1953, p. 647.

165[d] Talk before the American Historical Association, December 1954.

165[e] "Ego Development and Historical Change," p. 389.

166[a] *Childhood and Society,* p. 359.

166[b] *Ibid.,* pp. 244, 247, 251-2. Erikson makes some astute comments on the American Puritan tradition. He is on more doubtful ground when he attempts to correlate specific social institutions with specific psychological traits. He does not take adequately into consideration the different psychological needs which economic, political, or religious institutions can meet to some extent interchangeably, or with different emphases, at different historical periods. Similarly, his discussion of certain traits discovered among persons in Germany and Russia are interesting as descriptions of constellations of human characteristics rather than as attributes of national character.

166[c] See, for example, G. H. Mead, *Mind, Self & Society.*

166[d] See Gordon W. Allport, "The Ego in Contemporary Psychology," *Psychological Review,* Vol. 50, No. 5, Sept. 1943, pp. 451-78.

167[a] See, for example, Gardner Murphy, *Introduction to Psychology* and *Personality,* throughout; Urie Bronfenbrenner, "Toward an Integrated Theory of Personality," p. 253; Florence Kluckhohn, "Dominant and Variant Value Orientations," in Kluckhohn and Murray, *Personality in Nature, Society, and Culture,* p. 343; McClelland, *Personality,* p. 69; Angyal, *Foundations for a Science of Personality,* p. 200; Henry A. Murray, "Toward a Classification of Interaction," pp. 436-7.

167[b] For example, Hartmann speaks of "another set of functions we attribute to the ego [that] we call a person's character." ("Ego Psychology and the Problem of Adaptation," p. 385 n. 71.)

167[c] William James, *The Principles of Psychology,* Holt, 1890, Vol. I, Chap. X.

167[d] For example, Gardner Murphy, "Approaches to Personality," in M. H. Marx, *Psychological Theory,* pp. 522-5.

167[e] For example, McClelland, *Personality,* p. 529, and Jerome Bruner, "Personality Dynamics and the Process of Perceiving," in Blake and Ramsey, *Perception: An Approach to Personality,* p. 143 n.

167[f] For example, Angyal, *Foundations for a Science of Personality,* p. 118; Asch, *Social Psychology,* pp. 277-8; David P. Ausubel, *Ego Development and the Personality Disorders,* Grune and Stratton, 1952, p. '13.

168[a] *Ego Psychology and the Psychoses,* pp. 94-5. Cf. Hartmann's stress on the relative independence of ego development and its varied functions, particularly that of adaptation. ("Ego Psychology and the Problem of Adaptation," p. 380 and throughout.)

168[b] "Toward an Integrated Theory of Personality," pp. 222-3. Erikson notes that he uses identity to refer to what has been called the self by a number of investigators (self-concept by G. H. Mead, self-system or self-dynamism by Sullivan, fluctuating self-experience by Schilder and Federn, self-representation by Hartmann). ("The Problem of Ego Identity," pp. 102-05.)

169[a] Ortega y Gasset, "In Search of Goethe from Within," *Partisan Review,* Vol. 16, No. 12, Dec. 1949, pp. 1167-8.

169[b] Cf. Jones' discussion of Freud's development of the concept of the superego in *Sigmund Freud,* Vol. III, pp. 302-08.

170[a] Cf. Munroe, *Schools of Psychoanalytic Thought*, pp. 171-2, 273-6, 326, 329.

170[b] J. C. Flügel, *Man, Morals, and Society*, International Universities Press, 1945, p. 77; McClelland, *Personality*, p. 572. Alexander and Flügel think that it is best to keep the term superego for the more unconscious and irrational elements and ego-ideal for the more conscious and adaptable ones. This seems to me a distinction hard to maintain, and one that loses sight of some of the genetic and dynamic factors in the formation of the self- or ego-ideal. (Alexander, *Fundamentals of Psychoanalysis*, pp. 82-3.)

170[c] Carl Jung, *Collected Papers on Analytical Psychology*, Moffat Yard, 1917; *The Integration of the Personality*, Farrar and Rinehart, 1939; *Modern Man in Search of a Soul*, Harcourt, Brace, 1950.

170[d] "The *persona* is formed partly consciously as we develop specific personal ideals, goals, and a sense of our social role. Partly the process is unconscious as we identify with persons of importance to us and subtly take over the social values of our environment." (*Schools of Psychoanalytic Thought*, p. 558.)

170[e] Karen Horney, *Neurotic Personality of Our Time*, Norton, 1937; *New Ways in Psychoanalysis*, Norton, 1939; *Self-Analysis*, Norton, 1942; *Our Inner Conflicts*, Norton, 1945; *Neurosis and Human Growth*, Norton, 1950. Cf. Munroe, *Schools of Psychoanalytic Thought*, pp. 264-5, 366, 460-2, 533.

170[f] See, for example, Theodore R. Sarbin, "Role Theory," in Gardner Lindsey, ed., *Handbook of Social Psychology*, Addison-Wesley, 1954, Vol. I, pp. 224-5. Also S. Stansfeld Sargent, "Role and Ego in Psychology," in John H. Rohrer and Muzafer Sherif, *Social Psychology at the Crossroads*, Harper, 1951, p. 367.

170[g] Rapaport, *Organization and Pathology of Thought*, pp. 724-5.

172[a] Harry Hoijer, "The Sapir-Whorf Hypothesis," in Harry Hoijer, ed., *Language in Culture*, The American Anthropological Association, Vol. 56, No. 6, Part 2, Memoir No. 79, Dec. 1954, pp. 93-5. Hoijer makes it clear that the Sapir-Whorf hypothesis includes in language both its structural and its semantic aspects, *i.e.*, both its form and meaning.

Approaches to the study of language similar in some respects to that of the Sapir-Whorf hypothesis have been made by European scholars as far back as Herder—including Alexander von Humboldt, Ernst Cassirer, Johann Leo Weisgerber, Jost Trier, Jean Piaget, and L. Wittgenstein. (*Ibid.*, p. 93.)

172[b] David G. Mandelbaum, ed., *Selected Writings of Edward Sapir in Language, Culture and Personality*, University of California Press, 1949, p. 162.

172[c] *Ibid.*, p. 11.

172[d] *Ibid.*, pp. 10-11.

173[a] "Language, Mind, and Reality," *Etc., A Review of General Semantics,* Vol. X, No. 3, Spring 1952, pp. 173-4, 180, 182.

173[b] "An American Indian Model of the Universe," in John B. Carroll, ed., *Language, Thought, and Reality: Selected Writings of Benjamin Lee Whorf,* The Technology Press of Massachusetts Institute of Technology and John Wiley, 1956, p. 59.

174[a] *Ibid.,* p. 63. Cf. Hoijer's analysis of Navaho language and culture as illustrating the Sapir-Whorf hypothesis. ("The Sapir-Whorf Hypothesis," pp. 100-05.)

174[b] "Being and Value in a Primitive Culture."

174[c] "Linguistic Reflection of Wintu Thought," *International Journal of American Linguistics,* Vol. X, No. 4, Oct. 1944, pp. 182, 181.

174[d] "Notes on the Conception of Self Among the Wintu Indians," *Journal of Abnormal and Social Psychology,* Vol. 45, No. 3, July 1950. Maslow notes that in English we have a conjunction, *and,* to express the joining of two discrete entities but no conjunction to express the joining of two entities that are not discrete, but when joined form a unit, not a duality. (*Motivation and Personality,* p. 61 n.)

174[e] Strauss, *An Essay on Identity,* pp. 11, 17, 79-80, 92-4, 110, 128-9, 203-04.

175[a] Lewis S. Feuer, "Sociological Aspects of the Relation Between Language and Philosophy," *Philosophy of Science,* Vol. 20, No. 2, Apr. 1953, p. 90.

175[b] *Ibid.,* pp. 86 and 95.

175[c] *Ibid.,* pp. 95, 97.

176[a] Joshua Whatmough, *Language: A Modern Synthesis,* St. Martin's Press, 1956, pp. 224-7.

176[b] Graham Hough, review of A. J. Ayer's *Language, Truth, and Logic, New Statesman and Nation,* Apr. 5, 1947.

177[a] Iredell Jenkins, "Logical Positivism, Critical Idealism, and the Concept of Man," *Journal of Philosophy,* Vol. XLVII, No. 24, Nov. 23, 1950, pp. 677-95. Jenkins links Cassirer as a critical idealist with the logical positivists in impoverishing the concept of man in relation to the world.

177[b] The confusion that can arise from the use of the word symbol when what is meant is clearly sign is illustrated in George A. Miller's *Language and Communication* (McGraw-Hill, 1951). One chapter is entitled "*Rules* for Using Symbols" (pp. 100-18, italics mine). It includes the questions "How can redundancy be weeded out of a language?" and "Why do people tolerate such ambiguity?" and the subtitle "Language Engineering." Miller says of Basic English that it is "an interesting attempt to take advantage of the statistical aspects of language" (p. 115).

177[c] Cassirer, *Essay on Man,* p. 32. See also his *The Philosophy of Symbolic Forms,* Yale University Press, 1953, Vol. I, *Language.*

177[d] *Essay on Man,* p. 31.
177[e] *Ibid.,* p. 36.
178[a] Carl Jung, *Psychological Types,* Routledge and Kegan Paul, 1923, p. 601 and throughout. See also Munroe, *Schools of Psychoanalytic Thought,* pp. 549-52, 572-4. Cf. H. Flanders Dunbar's discussion of medieval symbolism as "that expression of meaningful experience which has basis in an association neither extrinsic arbitrary, nor intrinsic remaining in the realm of sense comparison, but intrinsic as expressing and reaching out toward the supersensible," a means by which the mind expresses those ideas "which it has not yet mastered." (*Symbolism in Medieval Thought,* Yale University Press, 1929, pp. 11, 13.)
178[b] Alfred North Whitehead, *Symbolism,* Macmillan, 1927, pp. 8 and 12.
178[c] *Language,* p. 8.
178[d] *Ibid.,* p. 12.
178[e] *Ibid.,* pp. 70-1.
178[f] *Ibid.,* p. 198.
178[g] *Ibid.,* p. 93.
178[h] *Ibid.,* p. 105.
178[i] *Ibid.,* p. 95.
179[a] Schilder, *Mind: Perception and Thought,* p. 247.
179[b] Kurt R. Eissler, "Limitations to the Psychotherapy of Schizophrenia," *Psychiatry,* Vol. 6, No. 4, Nov. 1943, pp. 383-4.
180[a] "The Effect of Brain Damage on the Personality," pp. 248-9. Cf. *The Organism,* pp. 310-11, 317, 392, and Piers and Singer, *Shame and Guilt.*
180[b] See, for example, criticisms in Rapaport, *Organization and Pathology of Thought,* p. 641, n. 149; p. 644, n. 153.
180[c] Alfred Korzybski, *Science and Sanity: An Introduction to Non-Aristotelian Systems and General Semantics,* 2nd ed., International Non-Aristotelian Library, 1941, pp. xx-xxii. Cf. Allport's protest against reductionism in the use of language, in "Emphasis on Molar Problems," pp. 166-8.
180[d] "Language in the Perceptual Process," in Blake and Ramsey, *Perception: An Approach to Personality,* p. 176, quoting Edward Sapir. (Cf. Lynd, *England in the Eighteen-Eighties,* Chap. III, and Meerloo, *Conversation and Communication,* pp. 31-2, on the putting together of different identities in a metaphor or a symbol.)
181[a] Korzybski, "Language in the Perceptual Process," pp. 177, 195-6.
183[a] Cf. Robert K. Merton's use of "theories of the middle range" which are "intermediate to the minor working hypotheses [of] . . . day-by-day . . . research, and the all-inclusive speculations comprising a master conceptual scheme from which it is hoped to derive a very large number of empirically observed uniformities of social behavior" (*Social Theory and Social Structure,* p. 5) and Urie Bronfenbrenner's

use of "intermediate hypotheses," which do not meet the requirements of rigorous experiment but have value in differentiating and organizing perception ("Toward an Integrated Theory of Personality," p. 210).

186[a] See, for example, Tolman, "A Psychological Model," pp. 349-50.

187[a] Howard Swiggert, *The Strong Box,* Houghton Mifflin, 1955, p. 81.

187[b] Samuel Stouffer, *et al., The American Soldier,* Vol. I, pp. 389-90.

188[a] Wayne Phillips, "Reforms by Marines Fail to End Charges of Training Abuses," New York *Times,* Feb. 12, 1957.

189[a] John Kenneth Galbraith, *American Capitalism: The Concept of Countervailing Power,* Houghton Mifflin, 1952, p. 69.

189[b] Whyte, *The Organization Man.* Cf. C. Wright Mills, *The Power Elite,* Oxford University Press, 1956.

189[c] *The Organization Man,* p. 394.

189[d] *Ibid.,* p. 395.

189[e] *Ibid.,* pp. 396-7.

190[a] See Robert S. Lynd, "The Middletown Spirit," in Robert S. and Helen Merrell Lynd, *Middletown in Transition,* Harcourt, Brace, 1937, pp. 402-86.

190[b] "Administrative Contributions to Democratic Character Formation at the Adolescent Level," in Kluckhohn and Murray, *Personality in Nature, Society, and Culture,* p. 665.

191[a] Quoted from L. Binswanger in Weigert, "Existentialism and Its Relation to Psychotherapy," p. 402.

191[b] Cf. Josef Nuttin's discussion of the combination of the privacy and penetrability of human consciousness involved in the sense of shame. ("Intimacy and Shame in the Dynamic Structure of Personality," in Martin L. Reymert, *Feelings and Emotions,* p. 344.)

In extreme form, detachment, role-playing, may lead beyond adjustment to pathology. "In the major neuroses, impaired reflective awareness is indicated by lack of insight . . . and special phenomena, such as states of depersonalization, multiple personalities, loss of personal identity, and amnesia." (Rapaport, *Organization and Pathology of Thought,* p. 706.)

192[a] Edmund Wilson, *Classics and Commercials,* Farrar, Straus, 1950, pp. 212-13, 211.

"The pleasure of Huxley's early novels," says Pritchett, came not from his people but "from the non-stop talk by which he drove them into exhaustion and nagged them into nothingness . . . he talked the clothes and souls off his people, he talked them out of life into limbo. . . . *Limbo* was the title of his first book of short stories. . . . In general his stories are not about people and situations, they are talk about people in relation to ideas that appear to have been set up in order to snub them. . . . No one drops so surprisingly into cliché when describing the ordinary run of feeling. . . . The effect is funny, cruel, devastating, indignant and dismissive . . . we are skillfully given an intellectual comedy—but not the *comédie humaine.*" (V. S. Pritchett, "Mellifluous Educator," review of Aldous Huxley, *Collected Short Stories,* Chatto and Windus, 1957, in the *New Statesman and Nation,* June 22, 1957.)

192[b] Edmund Wilson, "Ernest Hemingway: Bourdon Gauge of Morale," *Atlantic Monthly,* Vol. 164, July 1939.

192[c] "Books in General," *New Statesman and Nation,* Aug. 4, 1951.

192[d] "New Yorker Fiction," *The Nation,* Apr. 11, 1942.

193[a] Malcolm Cowley, "What Are the Qualities That Make an Author 'Modern'?" New York *Herald Tribune Book Review,* July 27, 1952.

194[a] Max Horkheimer, *The Eclipse of Reason,* Oxford University Press, 1947.

197[a] *Principles of Intensive Psychotherapy* and articles in *Psychiatry.*

197[b] *Schools of Psychoanalytic Thought,* pp. 326, 518.

198[a] *The Rape of the Mind.*

198[b] *Ibid.,* pp. 23-4.

198[c] *Ibid.,* p. 68.

198[d] *Ibid.,* p. 150.

198[e] *Battle for the Mind,* especially Chap. 4 and pp. 188-92.

198[f] Cf. Anselm Strauss' statement that in all these situations—religious or political conversion or therapy—"the learner has something to unlearn, to cope with, or as the psychoanalysts say, 'to work through.'" (*An Essay on Identity,* p. 165.)

199[a] Sargant, *Battle for the Mind,* p. 181 and throughout.

200[a] *Ibid.,* pp. 51, 55-7.

200[b] *Ibid.,* pp. 57-8, 167.

200[c] *Ibid.,* p. 51.

200[d] *Ibid.,* p. 55.

200[e] *Ibid.,* pp. 57-8.

200[f] *Ibid.,* pp. 59-60, 145, 153, 188-91, and throughout.

202[a] *Escape from Freedom* and *Man for Himself.* Fromm's next two books, *Psychoanalysis and Religion* (Yale University Press, 1950) and *The Forgotten Language* (Rinehart, 1951), are less concerned with the extent to which man is a social being and with the social factors in personality development. *The Sane Society* (Rinehart, 1955) returns to interest in the social environment. *The Art of Loving* (Harper, 1956) is chiefly concerned with the individual. Cf. the writings of Karen Horney and Harry Stack Sullivan previously cited.

202[b] *Eros and Civilization,* p. 245.

202[c] *Ibid.,* p. 246.

202[d] *Ibid.,* p. 257.

202[e] *Ibid.,* pp. 265-6.

204[a] "The Problem of Ego Identity," p. 57. Cf. Erving Goffman's use of self, ". . . I have implicitly been using a double definition of self:

the self as an image pieced together from the expressive implications of the full flow of events in an undertaking; and the self as a kind of player in a ritual game who copes honorably or dishonorably." ("On Face-Work," p. 225.)

Max Scheler also describes the "I" as a "double antithesis" between the outer world and the thou. (Alfred Schuetz, "Scheler's Theory of Inter-subjectivity," in "Symposium on the Significance of Max Scheler for Philosophy and Social Science," *Philosophy and Phenomenological Research*, Vol. II, No. 3, Mar. 1952, p. 325.)

204[b] Cf. Emily Dickinson's ways of describing the self: "The 'self' she variously designates . . . as the 'undiscovered continent' and the 'indestructible estate.' The solitudes of space, of the sea, even of death, she styles popular assemblies compared to 'That polar privacy —a soul admitted to itself.' " (Thomas H. Johnson, *Emily Dickinson*, Harvard University Press, 1955, p. 247.)

205[a] "Growth and Crises of the 'Healthy Personality,' " p. 189; *Childhood and Society*, p. 233.

205[b] "On the Sense of Inner Identity," p. 352.

206[a] "Growth and Crises of the 'Healthy Personality,' " pp. 188-9.

206[b] "The Problem of Ego Identity," pp. 70-1.

206[c] The chart expressing diagrammatically these eight stages of development is presented most fully in "The Problem of Ego Identity," p. 75.

206[d] *Ibid.*, pp. 70-1.

207[a] *Childhood and Society*, p. 223.

207[b] *Ibid.*, pp. 360-3, and "The Problem of Ego Identity."

211[a] *A Writer's Diary*, pp. 324-5. Cf. Handlin's statement that in the Old Country "this house in this village, these fields by these trees . . . had testified to the peasant's *I*, had fixed his place in the visible universe." (*The Uprooted*, p. 105.)

212[a] Cf. Nuttin's statement that "The greater the distance between the . . . raw materials . . . of human nature and the ideals incorporated in cultural behavior, the greater the task to be performed by the process of personality integration." (Josef Nuttin, "Intimacy and Shame in the Dynamic Structure of Personality," in Martin L. Reymert, *Feelings and Emotions*, p. 349.)

212[b] Kingsley Davis, "Mental Hygiene and the Class Structure," pp. 378-9.

213[a] *Conceptions of Modern Psychiatry*, p. 87. See also Sullivan's *The Interpersonal Theory of Psychiatry*.

213[b] *Conceptions of Modern Psychiatry*, p. 97, n. 66.

213[c] *Ibid.* Sullivan made it clear that he regarded reactionary conservatives as well as radical Utopians—in contrast to rational liberals—as persons who take extreme positions as a result of disturbance in interpersonal relations.

214[a] "Ego Development and Historical Change," pp. 388-9.

214[b] *Eros and Civilization.*

215[a] President Eisenhower, when he was President of Columbia University before he became President of the United States, said this. (New York *Herald Tribune,* Mar. 12, 1951.)

216[a] David Garnett, *The Golden Echo,* Harcourt, Brace, 1954, Vol. I, pp. 59-61.

216[b] The damaging effect upon children of hypocritical or counterfeit attitudes of their parents is widely recognized. See, for example, Phyllis Greenacre, "Conscience in the Psychopath," *American Journal of Orthopsychiatry,* Vol. 15, No. 3, July 1945, pp. 495-509, and Sullivan's discussions in his various works cited.

217[a] *King Lear,* V, iii, 30-2. We may regard Edmund as primarily a double-dealing villain who almost to the last allowed no human feeling to deter him from his evil course, or as a necessary instrument of history whose very ruthlessness helped to destroy an outworn past and thus make way for the future. In either case, the problem posed by his version of realism remains.

217[b] *Ibid.,* V, iii, 32-3.

218[a] *Ibid.,* V, i, 68-9.

218[b] Cf. J. Glenn Gray, "The Idea of Death in Existentialism," *The Journal of Philosophy,* Vol. XLVIII, No. 5, Mar. 1, 1951, p. 114.

218[c] Unselective response to reality or to other persons appears to depend less on sensitivity to others, more on a weak sense of self; less on heightened sensitivity to external stimuli, more on lowered sensitivity to internal stimuli. (Elaine Bell, "Inner-directed and Other-directed attitudes," Ph.D. dissertation, Yale University.)

219[a] See Helen M. Lynd, "Realism and the Intellectual in a Time of Crisis," *The American Scholar,* Vol. 21, No. 1, Winter 1951-1952.

220[a] Account in the New York *Times,* Sept. 9, 1954, of the meeting of the World Council of Churches in Evanston, Illinois, Sept. 1954.

221[a] *The Rape of the Mind,* p. 154.

221[b] Alan Moorehead, *The Traitors: The Double Life of Fuchs, Pontecorvo and Nunn May,* Hamish Hamilton, 1952.

222[a] "The Age of Treason," *The New Statesman and Nation,* July 26, 1952.

222[b] "Books in General," a review of Franz Borkenau, *European Communism,* Faber, 1953, *New Statesman and Nation,* June 6, 1953.

222[c] *Ibid.*

222[d] Review, July 26, 1952.

223[a] Freud, *Reflections on War and Death,* Moffat Yard, 1918, pp. 13-14.

223[b] Morton Grodzins, *The Loyal and the Disloyal: Social Boundaries of Patriotism and Treason,* University of Chicago Press, 1956.

223[c] *Ibid.,* pp. 106, 110-20.

223[d] *Ibid.,* p. 135. Grodzins does not ignore the different character of disloyalty in a totalitarian and in a democratic society. He also points out explicitly the ways in which personal insecurities may contribute to making a traitor; but he does not think that personality factors alone are decisive. (*Ibid.*, pp. 171, 189, 202.)

223[e] *Ibid.*, pp. 131, 135, 192.

224[a] *Ibid.*, pp. 205, 210, 213.

224[b] Rebecca West's *Meaning of Treason* (Viking, 1947), for example, takes this naïve view.

224[c] *The Rape of the Mind*, p. 237. See also pp. 253, 260, 262, 279, 288, 303, and Chap. 14.

225[a] Murray Kempton, "Robert Oppenheimer and the Iron Circle," *The Progressive*, Sept. 1954.

225[b] See A. J. Liebling's discussion of this problem in his review of *The Witness, The New Yorker*, Nov. 19, 1949.

225[c] Victor Serge, *The Case of Comrade Tulayev*, Hamish Hamilton, 1951.

226[a] Erikson comments that many Americans find it difficult to stand the tension demanded by polarities in American culture, "the never-ceasing necessity of remaining tentative in order to be free to take the next step, to turn the next corner." ("Ego Development and Historical Change," pp. 388-9.)

226[b] Jean Marie Guyau, *A Sketch of Morality Independent of Obligation or Sanction*, Watts, pp. 210-11, 91. Cf. Muriel Rukeyser's statement that Melville and Whitman had to do with the expression of the possible—the necessary, *because* it was possible. (*Willard Gibbs*, Doubleday, 1942, p. 363.)

228[a] Letter to George and Georgiana Keats, Feb., Mar., Apr., 1819. Maurice Buxton Forman, ed., *The Letters of John Keats*, Oxford University Press, 1931, Vol. II, pp. 361-4.

229[a] "The Development of Focal Attention," p. 320.

229[b] *Ibid.*

230[a] *Ibid.*, p. 313.

230[b] The self-ideal is also sometimes used to include the prohibiting aspects of the superego, Horney's derogatory view of a romanticized self-ideal, and the incorporation of prescribed social roles.

232[a] *Anna Karenina*, p. 168.

233[a] Adolescents in our society frequently go through difficulties of "role diffusion," a taking over of a variety of cultural roles in an attempt to find in them a confirmation of, or even a substitute for, inner design. (Erikson, *Childhood and Society*, pp. 227-8.)

234[a] Barker Fairley, *A Study of Goethe*, p. 231.

234[b] See Erikson, "The Dream Specimen of Psychoanalysis," in Knight and Friedman, *Psychoanalytic Psychiatry and Psychology*, Vol. I, p. 169.

235[a] *Conceptions of Modern Psychiatry*, p. 47.

235[b] See, for example, "The Illusion of Personal Individuality," *Psychiatry*, Vol. 13, No. 3, Aug. 1950.

235[c] *Middlemarch*, pp. 187-91.

235[d] *Chance*.

237[a] Marx and Engels, *The German Ideology*, pp. 74-8 and p. 58, and "Alienated Labor."

237[b] Harold Rosenberg, "The Pathos of the Proletariat," *Kenyon Review*, Vol. XI, No. 4, Autumn 1949, pp. 610, 611-13.

239[a] E. M. Forster, "Proust," in *Abinger Harvest*, Harcourt, Brace, 1936, p. 100.

239[b] Cf. Erikson, "The Problem of Ego Identity," pp. 80-83, 118.

239[c] *Nicomachean Ethics*, Book IV, Chap. 9.

240[a] *Macbeth*, V, ii, 19-20.

240[b] *Ibid.*, III, iv, 24-5.

240[c] *Richard II*, V, i, 66-7.

240[d] *Venus and Adonis*, 803.

241[a] Goldstein, "The Effect of Brain Damage on the Personality," p. 251; cf. *The Organism*, pp. 317, 392, and Piers and Singer, *Shame and Guilt*, pp. 11, 16.

241[b] Weigert, "Existentialism and Its Relation to Psychotherapy," p. 405.

243[a] Aaron Copland, *What to Listen for in Music*, Mentor Books, 1939.

244[a] Cf. also Max Wertheimer, "On Truth," *Social Research*, Vol. I, No. 2, May 1934.

244[b] Rudolf Arnheim, "The Priority of Expression," *The Journal of Aesthetics and Art Criticism*, Vol. VIII, No. 2, Dec. 1949.

244[c] See Helen M. Lynd, "An Undiscovered Language," *The Nation*, May 31, 1952.

245[a] Joseph Kahnweiler, *Juan Gris*, Curt Valentin, 1947, p. 65.

245[b] *Ibid.*, p. 77.

245[c] Leo Spitzer, "Perspectivism in 'Don Quijote'" in *Linguistics and Literary History*, Princeton University Press, 1948, pp. 56 and 72. Cf. also Spitzer's "Milieu and Ambiance: An Essay in Historical Semantics," *Philosophy and Phenomenological Research*, Vol. III, No. 1, Sept. 1942.

246[a] William Empson, *Seven Types of Ambiguity*, Chatto and Windus, 1949 and his *The Structure of Complex Words*. See also W. H. Clemen, *The Development of Shakespeare's Imagery*, Methuen, 1951, pp. 90-1.

246[b] Quoted in Patrick Heron, review of Kahnweiler's *Juan Gris*, *New Statesman and Nation*, Mar. 20, 1948.

246[c] Jacques Hadamard, *The Psychology of Invention in the Mathematical Field*, Princeton University Press, 1945, pp. 65 ff.

246[d] *Ibid.*, pp. 77, 95-6.

247[a] *Ex-prodigy*, pp. 212-13.

247[b] Schachtel, "Memory and Childhood Amnesia," pp. 3-49.
247[c] *Ibid.*, p. 9.
248[a] *Ibid.*, pp. 12-13.
248[b] *Ibid.*, p. 20.
248[c] *Ibid.*, p. 44.
249[a] James Joyce, *Stephen Hero,* Modern Library, pp. 146-7.
251[a] This is the water color "The Crucifixion" of 1801.
252[a] J. Glenn Gray, "The Idea of Death in Existentialism," p. 114. This is Gray's summary of the existentialist view, not his own.
252[b] See Lasswell, *Power and Personality,* pp. 98-9; Fromm, *Escape from Freedom,* especially pp. 179-85; Virgil C. Aldrich, "An Ethics of Shame," *International Journal of Ethics,* Vol. L, No. 1, Oct. 1939, p. 62.
252[c] See Lee in "Greece," p. 81. The conceptions of pride and humility as essential to each other and of the embracing of multiple possibilities as essential for freedom have deep roots in human history. In primitive ceremonies connected with fertility and initiation there is heightened performance of *both* eating and cleansing. In the transition from tribal to political society in Greece, about the sixth or seventh centuries, these two experiences were torn apart; the ritual of Dionysus with sacred intoxication and the devouring of an animal and the ritual of Apollo with emphasis on cleansing, asceticism, or at least moderation, were separated. Mental illness tends to concentrate on one aspect of life—fertility *or* abnegation, eating *or* cleansing. In mental health these complementary aspects of life cannot be wrenched apart; contradiction and multiple possibilities must be entertained. Multiplicity and variation are of its essence.
253[a] *Othello,* I, iii, 314-15.
254[a] *Middlemarch,* pp. 401-02.
256[a] "The Dynamic Perception and the Symbolism of Form," p. 85.
256[b] Cf. Meredith, *An Essay on Comedy;* Burke, *Attitudes Toward History,* Vol. I, p. 96; Loewenberg, Introduction, *Hegel Selections,* Scribner's, 1929; Hegel, *Phenomenology of Mind.*
257[a] Loewenberg, *Hegel Selections,* pp. xxvii-viii.
257[b] *Ibid.,* xxxiv-v, xxxvii. Cf. Kenneth Burke's statement that "all the issues with which we have been concerned come to a head in the problem of identity. Bourgeois naturalism in its most naive manifestation made a blunt distinction between 'individual' and 'environment,' hence leading automatically to the notion that an individual's 'identity' is something private, peculiar to himself. And when bourgeois psychologists . . . discovered . . . that a man 'identifies himself' with all sorts of manifestations beyond himself . . . they set about trying to 'cure' him of this tendency." (*Attitudes Toward History,* Vol. II, pp. 138-9.)
257[c] Job 9:19 and 21 (Jastrow translation).
257[d] Job 13:15.

Acknowledgments

The author wishes to thank the following for permission to quote material from the books and articles listed:

American Book Company: Kurt Goldstein, *The Organism.*

American Psychological Association: Dorothy Lee in *Journal of Abnormal and Social Psychology,* "The Conception of Self Among the Wintu Indians" (Vol. 45, July, 1950) and "Are Basic Needs Ultimate?" (Vol. 32, 1948).

American Psychological Review: O. H. Mowrer, "Stimulus-Response Theory of Anxiety."

Appleton-Century-Crofts, Inc.: Boris Sidis, *The Psychology of Laughter.*

Edward Arnold (Publishers), Ltd.: E. M. Forster, *A Passage to India.*

Basic Books, Inc.: Paul Federn, *Ego Psychology and the Psychoses.*

Cambridge University Press: D'Arcy Thompson, *On Growth and Form.*

Jonathan Cape, Ltd.: Rebecca West, *The Harsh Voice;* Sigmund Freud, *Civilization and Its Discontents.*

Chatto and Windus, Ltd.: Sigmund Freud, *Collected Papers;* F. R. Leavis, *Mill on Bentham and Coleridge.*

Columbia University Press: David Rapaport, *Organization and Pathology of Thought;* Paul Schilder, *Goals and Desires of Man* and *Mind: Perception and Thought in Their Constructive Aspects.*

J. M. Dent & Sons, Ltd.: Joseph Conrad, *Chance;* David Hume, *Treatise on Human Nature* (Everyman edition).

Doubleday & Company, Inc.: George Madden Martin, *Emmy Lou, Her Book and Her Heart;* W. Somerset Maugham, *Of Human Bondage* (Modern Library edition).

E. P. Dutton & Co., Inc.: Everyman's Library Series, David Hume, *Treatise on Human Nature.*

The Dryden Press, Inc.: Ruth L. Munroe, *Schools of Psychoanalytic Thought.*

Faber and Faber, Ltd.: T. S. Eliot, *Selected Essays,* "The Metaphysical Poets."

Farrar, Straus and Cudahy, Inc.: Ward Moore, *Bring the Jubilee;* Edmund Wilson, *Classics and Commercials.*

Grune & Stratton, Inc.: Grace Rubin-Rabson, tr., Marguerite Sechehaye, *Autobiography of a Schizophrenic Girl.*

Harcourt, Brace & Co., Inc.: E. M. Forster, *A Passage to India;* Virginia Woolf, *A Writer's Diary* and *Night and Day.*

Harper & Brothers: George Eliot, *Mill on the Floss* (Harper edition); Thomas Hardy, *The Return of the Native;* A. H. Maslow, *Motivation and Personality.*

Harvard University Press: Kurt Goldstein, *Human Nature in the Light of Psychopathology;* Talcott Parsons and Edward A. Shils, *Toward a General Theory of Action.*

Hogarth Press: Sigmund Freud, *Outline of Psycho-Analysis;* Virginia Woolf, *A Writer's Diary* and *Night and Day.*

Henry Holt & Co., Inc.: Lancelot L. Whyte, *The Next Development in Man.*

Houghton Mifflin Company: John Kenneth Galbraith, *American Capitalism: The Concept of Countervailing Power;* Carson McCullers, *The Member of the Wedding;* Howard Swiggert, *The Strong Box.*

International Journal of American Linguistics: Dorothy Lee, "Linguistic Reflection of Wintu Thought" (October, 1944).

International Society for General Semantics: Benjamin Whorf and Harry Hoijer, "Language, Mind, and Reality," in *ETC* (Spring, 1952).

International Psychological Association: David Rapaport, "Paul Schilder's Contribution to the Theory of Thought," in *International Journal of Psychoanalysis* (XXXII, 1951).

International Publishers: Karl Marx and Friedrich Engels, *The German Ideology.*

International Universities Press, Inc.: Robert P. Knight and C. R. Friedman, *Psychoanalytic Psychiatry and Psychology;* Ernst Kris, *Psychoanalytic Explorations in Art.*

Journal of the American Psychoanalytic Association: Erik M. Erikson, "The Problem of Identity" (January, 1956).

Alfred A. Knopf, Inc.: Elizabeth Bowen, *Death of the Heart;* Clyde Kluckhohn and Henry A. Murray, *Personality in Nature, Society and Culture.*

Harold D. Lasswell: *World Politics and Personal Insecurity.*

Little, Brown & Company: Oscar Handlin, *The Uprooted;* Aileen Pippett, *The Moth and the Star.*

Liveright Publishing Corporation: Sigmund Freud, *Group Psychology and the Analysis of the Ego.*

Lund Humphries: Lancelot L. Whyte, *Aspects of Form.*

McGraw-Hill Book Company, Inc.: John Dollard and Neal E. Miller, *Personality and Psychotherapy.*

The Macmillan Company: Doestoevsky, *Short Novels* and *The Brothers Karamazov;* Radhakamal Mukerjee, *The Social Structure of Values;* Turgenev, *A House of Gentlefolk.*

Thomas Nelson & Sons: Patrick Mullahy (ed.), *A Study of Interpersonal Relations.*

The New American Library of World Literature, Inc.: Margaret Mead (ed.), *Cultural Patterns and Technical Change.*

The New Republic: Kenneth Burke, *Attitudes Toward History.*

New Statesman: R. H. S. Crossman, "The Age of Reason," in *New Statesman and Nation* (July 26, 1952).

New York Herald Tribune: Malcolm Cowley, "What Are the Qualities That Make an Author 'Modern'?" *Book Review* (July 27, 1952).

New York Philosophical Library, Inc.: Jean-Paul Sartre, *Being and Nothingness.*

New York Times: Wayne Phillips, "Reforms by Marines Fail to End Charges of Training Abuses" (February 12, 1957).

W. W. Norton & Company, Inc.: Erik H. Erikson, *Childhood and Society;* Sigmund Freud, *Outline of Psychoanalysis;* Harold D. Lasswell, *Power and Personality;* Rainer Maria Rilke, *The Journey of My Other Self.*

Oxford University Press: R. G. Collingwood, *An Autobiography;* Maurice Burton Forman, *The Letters of John Keats;* F. O. Matthiessen, *The Achievement of T. S. Eliot;* Henry A. Murray, *Explorations in Personality.*

Pantheon Books, Inc.: Joseph Campbell, *The Hero with a Thousand Faces* (Bollingen Series, XVII).

Prentice-Hall, Inc.: Charles W. Morris, *Signs, Language, and Behavior.*

Princeton University Press: Jacques Hadamard, *The Psychology of Invention in the Mathematical Field;* Samuel A. Stouffer and Associates, *The American Soldier: Combat and Its Aftermath.*

Psychiatry: Erving Goffman, "On Face-Work" (Vol. 18, August, 1955); Kurt Goldstein, "Effect of Brain Damage on Personality" (Vol. 15, August, 1952); Ernest Schachtel, "The Dynamic Perception and the Symbolism of Form" (Vol. 4, February, 1941) and "The Development of Focal Attention" (Vol. 17, November, 1954); Edith Weigert, "Existentialism and Its Relation to Psychotherapy" (Vol. 7, November, 1949).

The Psychoanalytic Quarterly: Adelaide McF. Johnson, "Some Etiological Aspects of Repression, Guilt and Hostility" (Vol. XX, October, 1951).

Random House, Inc.: John Donne, *Complete Poetry and Selected Prose of John Donne;* Modern Library edition: Marcel Proust, *The Captive,* and Tolstoy, *Anna Karenina.*

Henry Regnery Company: Kurt Riezler, *Man: Mutable and Immutable.*

Charles Scribner's Sons: Jacob Loewenberg, *Hegel Selections.*

Martin Secker & Warburg, Ltd.: Franz Kafka, *The Trial;* Joshua Whatmough, *Language: A Modern Synthesis.*
Simon and Schuster, Inc.: William H. Whyte, Jr., *The Organization Man;* Norbert Wiener, *Ex-Prodigy: My Childhood and Youth.*
The Society of Authors: George Bernard Shaw, *Selected Prose.*
St. Martin's Press, Inc.: Joshua Whatmough, *Language: A Modern Synthesis.*
Charles C. Thomas: Gerhart Piers and Milton B. Singer, *Shame and Guilt.*
UNESCO: Tensions and Technology Series, Dorothy Lee, "Greece," in M. Mead (ed.), *Cultural Patterns and Technical Change.*
University of California Press: David C. Mandelbaum (ed.), *Selected Writings of Edward Sapir in Language, Culture and Personality.*
University of Chicago Press: Franz Alexander, *Dynamic Psychiatry.*
Viking Press, Inc.: Rebecca West, *The Harsh Voice.*
A. P. Watt: Doestoevsky, *The Brothers Karamazov;* William Sargant, *Battle for the Mind.*
John Wiley & Sons and the Technology Press of Massachusetts Institute of Technology: John B. Carroll (ed.), *Language, Thought, and Reality: Selected Writings of Benjamin Lee Whorf.*
World Publishing Company: Joost A. M. Meerloo, *The Rape of the Mind.*
Yale Review: Erik H. Erikson, "The First Psychoanalyst" (Vol. XLVI, September, 1946).
Yale University Press: Ernst Cassirer, *Essay on Man.*

Index